Anti-Inflammatory Diet Slow Cooker Cookbook

Ready-To-Go Recipes to Fight Inflammation, Preventing Disease and Stay Healthy

By Jane Kennedy

Copyrights©2019 By Jane Kennedy
All Rights Reserved

This document is geared towards providing exact and reliable information in regards to the topic and issue covered. The publication is sold with the idea that the publisher is not required to render accounting, officially permitted, or otherwise, qualified services. If advice is necessary, legal or professional, a practiced individual in the profession should be ordered.

Legal Notice: The book is copyright protected. This is only for personal use. You cannot amend, distribute, sell, use, quote or paraphrase any part or the content within this book without the consent of the author.

Under no circumstance will any legal responsibility or blame be held against the publisher for any reparation, damages, or monetary loss due to the information herein, either directly or indirectly.

Disclaimer Notice: Please note the information contained within this document is for educational and entertainment purpose only. Every attempt has been made to provide accurate, up to date and reliable complete information. No warranties of any kind are expressed or implied. Reader acknowledge that the author is not engaging in the rendering of legal, financial, medical or professional advice. The content of this book has been derived from various sources. Please consult a licensed professional before attempting any techniques outlined in this book.

Table of Content

Introduction 1
Chapter 1: Understanding Inflammation 3
    What Is Inflammation? 3
    Common Symptoms of Inflammation 4
    Health Risks of Inflammation 5
    Summary 6
Chapter 2: The Ultimate Anti-Inflammatory Diet Action Plan 7
    What is Anti-Inflammatory Diet 8
    Anti-Inflammatory Diet and Calorie Count 8
    Guidelines for Anti-inflammatory Diet 8
    General Tips for Anti-Inflammatory Diet 11
Chapter 3: Ultimate Guide to Use a Slow Cooker 12
    What is Slow Cooker, and How Does it Work? 13
    Understanding Slow Cooker Settings and Buttons 15
    Slow Cooker Accessories 15
    Cooking Hacks for Slow Cooker 16
Chapter 4: 63 Amazing Anti-Inflammatory Slow Cooker Recipes 18
Breakfast and Brunch 18
    Slow Cooker French toast Casserole 18
    Crackpot Banana Foster 19
    Chicken and Quinoa Burrito Bowl 20
    Nutty Blueberry Banana Oatmeal 21
    Slow Cooker Steamed Cinnamon Apples 22
    Carrot Rice with Scrambled Eggs 23
Salads 26
    Slow Cooker Chicken Romaine Salad 26
    Slow-Cooked Kale with Smashed Garlic & Red Onions 27

Slow Cooker Avocado Chicken Salad.. 28
Golden Tagine Crockpot Salad.. 29
Slow Cooker Warm 3-Bean Salad... 30
Curtido Cabbage Salad.. 31
Slow Cooker Hot German Potato Salad..32

Soups and Stews..34
Healthy Broccoli Curry Soup...34
Best Detox Lentil Soup..35
Broccoli Turmeric Soup...36
Seafood Ste.. 37
Slow Cooker Peasant Stew.. 38
Healthy Chicken Pot Pie Stew... 39

Appetizers and Snacks..41
Crockpot Baked Sweet Potatoes.. 41
Slow-Cooked Salsa.. 42
Crockpot Ginger Bread Latte... 43
Anti-Inflammatory Cauliflower Fried Rice... 44
Cranberry Poached Pears... 45
Slow Cooker Cheddar Polenta with Winter Greens.. 46

Vegetables and Vegan...48
Slow Cooker Vegan Gumbo.. 48
Slow Cooker Loaded Baked Potato Casserole..49
Slow Cooker Stuffed Bell Pepper.. 50
Slow Cooker Eggplant Lasagna... 51
Slow Cooker Ratatouille.. 52
Plant-Based Slow Cooker Chili... 53

Beans and Legumes...55
Slow Cooker Southern Style Green Beans.. 55
Slow Cooker Black Bean Soup for Two..56
Slow Cooker Red Lentil Curry.. 57
Slow Cooker Barbecue Beans..58
Sloppy Joes Made With Lentils... 60
Slow Cooker Spanish Style Chickpeas..61

    The Ultimate 9-Bean Slow Cooker Soup..62

Poultry and Meat...64
    Slow Cooker Turkey Chili...64
    Slow Cooker Black Bean and Chicken Chowder..65
    Slow Cooker Spinach Artichoke Chicken...66
    Healthy Slow Cooker Chicken Dumplings...67
    Turkey Sloppy Joes..68
    Greek Lemon Chicken...69
    Spinach-Chicken Meatball...70

Beef Lamb and Pork..72
    Korean Beef Lettuce Wraps...72
    Healthier Slow Cooker Texas Roadhouse Chili for Two..73
    Slow Cooker Pork Tenderloin..74
    Slow Cooker Moroccan Beef Stew..75
    5 –Ingredient BBQ Pulled Pork for Two..76
    Low Carb Beef Stroganoff...77

Fish and Seafood...79
    Slow Cooker Salmon with Creamy Lemon Sauce...79
    Orange-Chipotle Shrimp in Butter Lettuce Cups...81
    Crockpot Halibut Stew...82
    Slow Cooker Fish and Tomatoes..83
    Slow Cooker Italian Herb Salmon...84
    Healthy Slow Cooker Tuna Casserole...85

Desserts...87
    Slow Cooker Fudge...87
    Pumpkin Pecan Cobbler Recipe..88
    Slow Cooker Lemon Bars...89
    Slow Cooker Chocolate Peanut Butter Cake...90
    Slow Cooker Hot Fudge Cake...91
    Almond Rice Chia Pudding..92

Introduction

As a nutritionist, I understand how different the problems are of various people when it comes to their diet and lifestyle. Whenever someone comes to me for a diet plan for their weight issues or problems regarding other conditions, I ask them one thing, "Do you follow a balanced diet?" Unfortunately, most people do not follow a wholesome balanced diet and look forward to diets such as Keto, Gluten-free or Paleo to work wonders on their bodies. Although these diets have a fair share of benefits and can help with few medical conditions, they are not fit for everyone. If you are having weight issues and other problems related to your diet, you should check if you are following the proper diet.

However, there are a few conditions that need more than a balanced diet. In fact, there is a need to change the diet plan completely to treat some conditions regardless of how healthy a diet the patient claims to have. One such condition is excessive inflammation in one's body. Inflammation is a necessary process to prevent your body from developing infections and getting sick. But some people are naturally prone to excessive inflammation, i.e. their diet causes more inflammation, or they suffer from a disease that causes inflammation.

There is one thing common regarding the treatment of all three cases; taking care of the diet. Many foods that are supposed to be healthy are not good for people with inflammation issues. As a result, they need to consume anti-inflammatory foods.

Most anti-inflammatory foods are nutrient-rich plant-based foods. When you are on an anti-inflammatory diet, you have to avoid processed foods, sugary foods, and meats. Sounds too difficult? There are many anti-inflammatory foods around you that you usually eat. At first, it might seem that eating will become boring and less tasty when you cut down on certain foods. However, here are some mouth-watering slow-cooker recipes for you that you can prepare in no time to bring flavors back to your foods.

If you follow the recipes and diet plan in this book to reduce inflammation in your body, there are certain things for you to note.

Anti-inflammatory Recipes

The recipes and meal plan devised for you are purely based on the nutritional sciences of food. The foods that we will discuss have good anti-inflammatory and nutritional properties that will reduce excess inflammation. The recipes here are the perfect alternative to foods that cause inflammation.

Use of Slow Cooker

What makes this cookbook unique is that all the anti-inflammatory recipes are more or less specific for a slow cooker. Though there is no hard and fast rule for preparing anti-inflammatory recipes in a slow cooker, once you follow these recipes, you will see how super convenient it is for daily cooking and why it is the best choice for those on an anti-inflammatory diet. If you do not have a slow cooker, I recommend you get one. It does not cost you much and is an excellent investment when you are on a strict diet and a tight working schedule. If you are away from home and do not have a slow cooker available then follow the recipes with low cooking time, which you can easily make in any pot, pan, or wok available.

Consult Your Doctor

Consult your doctor and let them know that you are changing your meal plan. The dietary changes I am going to recommend are anything but dangerous. But a major change in your diet if you have an ongoing condition or especially if you are on medication can affect your health.For example, your blood sugar might fall too low, which is not good for you.

Ask your doctor whether changes in your meal plan with anti-inflammatory foods can go well with your medications or your conditions, especially if you have diabetes. Your doctor will advise you better and might stop or alter your medication.

Healthy Lifestyle Habits

Where adding anti-inflammatory rich foods in your diet can have an immense effect on your health, you should not be ignoring the basic healthy habits. Getting a good night sleep and drinking plenty of water sound unimportant; following them is crucial to maintain a healthy lifestyle. Drinking lots of water helps in reducing inflammation in your body. Goodnight sleep is essential for the proper functioning of your body. You need it to combat any health problems you are going through. Exercising is a great option to boost your metabolism and reduce inflammation.

Chapter 1: Understanding Inflammation

Before moving on to anti-inflammatory foods to reduce inflammation, it is necessary to understand what inflammation really is. In-depth knowledge about inflammation can help you treat it better and follow a diet plan that suits you best.

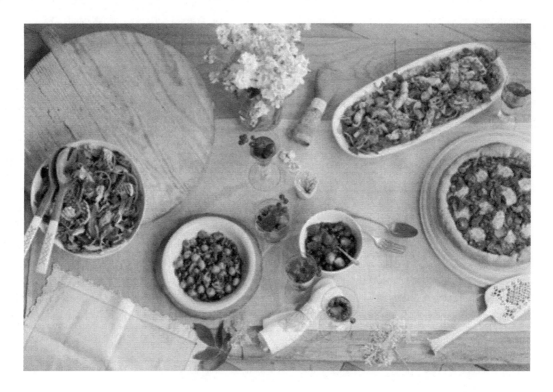

What Is Inflammation?

Inflammation is a process by which our body produces and releases specialized immune cells, mainly white blood cells in response to the invasion of foreign agents such as bacteria or viruses. Inflammation is an ongoing natural process, which prevents the development of infection in our bodies or fights off infections when they occur. Our body, in one way or the other, is undergoing inflammation most of the time without us knowing about it. Fever is also a result of inflammation – increasing the body's temperature to help fight off the foreign agents.

The problem arises when inflammation gets uncontrolled, or it occurs when there is no foreign agent infecting your body. There are conditions like Arthritis, which cause the immune system to release immune cells (white blood cells and cytokines), triggering an immune response and increasing the inflammation in the body. Some auto-immune diseases lead to misdirected inflammation. Following are the examples of autoimmune diseases:

- Type-1 Diabetes
- Rheumatoid Arthritis
- Psoriatic Arthritis
- Gouty Arthritis
- Multiple Sclerosis
- Inflammatory Bowel disease
- Addison's Disease
- Graves' Disease

Common Symptoms of Inflammation

Two people suffering from inflammation may not necessarily experience the same symptoms. However, following are the common symptoms seen in most cases of inflammation.

- Redness on skin
- Itching or rash
- Pain in chest
- Swollen Joints
- Swollen joints feeling warm when touched
- Pain in the joints
- Stiffness in the joint
- Loss of function in the joints

Redness and itchiness in the skin usually indicate skin allergies. Alone, these two symptoms do not signify inflammation. However, redness is the first visual symptom of inflammation. When inflammation occurs, the flow of blood to inflamed site increases, causing redness, heat, and swelling.

Arthritis is one of the most common causes of inflammation. Stiffness, pain, swelling, loss of function, or any other symptoms associated with joints is a clear indication of inflammation caused by arthritis.

In several cases, inflammation is also related to flu-like symptoms such as:
- Headaches
- Loss of appetite
- Tiredness and fatigue
- Weakness
- Fever
- Chills
- Loss of Appetite
- Stiffness in muscles

Health Risks of Inflammation

Now that you are aware of the symptoms of the inflammation, it is easier for you to understand its health effects and risks. To know about the risks of inflammation, it is better to understand its process.

During inflammation, there is secretion of the chemicals from the white blood cells into the blood or tissues to protect them from the foreign agent. The release of chemicals increases the blood flow causing redness, heating, and swelling of the inflamed site. The leak of some chemicals in the tissue can cause further swelling. This can stimulate the nerves and eventually cause pain.

The number of these blood cells and chemicals secretion in the joints leads to irritation and swelling. The swelling in the lining of the joints can damage the joints, causing the wearing of the cartilage. Cartilage is an important component of the bone that cushions the bone during movement and prevents the wear and tear.

Chronic inflammation can weaken and damage the bones, especially joints. There is no cure or remedy for damaged joints, but there are options for treatments such as knee-replacing operation.

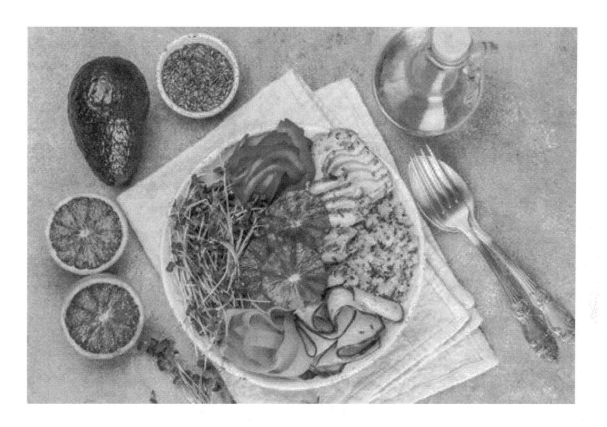

Summary

- ✓ Inflammation is the body's attempt to prevent or heal the body from infection. It is a necessary process to heal wounds and damaged tissues.
- ✓ Redness, swelling, and heating are common symptoms of inflammation.
- ✓ Chronic inflammation has harmful effects on the body and is caused by auto-immune conditions or diseases.
- ✓ Chronic inflammation can further cause severe diseases like Rheumatoid Arthritis, which can permanently damage the joints.

Chapter 2: The Ultimate Anti-Inflammatory Diet Action Plan

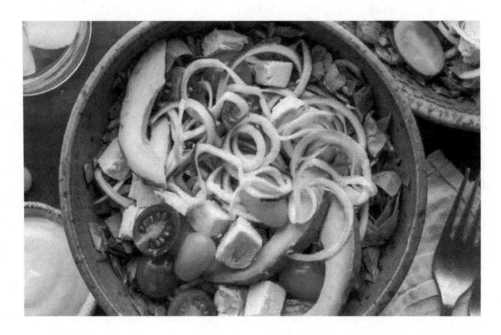

I cannot stress enough about how beneficial an anti-inflammatory diet is for your body. Your food choices determine the level of inflammation that takes place inside your body. An anti-inflammatory diet is effective for combating severe inflammation problems and for preventing the following conditions:

- Alzheimer's Disease
- Severe Allergies
- Cancer
- Depression
- PCOS for some women
- Inflammatory bowel disease
- Inflammatory bowel syndrome
- Crohn's Disease
- Stroke

To follow an anti-inflammatory diet, you don't necessarily have to suffer from chronic inflammation. An anti-inflammatory diet helps people treat problems such as obesity, slow metabolism, diabetes, feeling low and dull, and stress. Paired with proper sleep and regular exercise, an anti-inflammatory diet can do wonders for your body.

What is Anti-Inflammatory Diet

An anti-inflammatory diet is quite similar to a Mediterranean diet. Both emphasize on consuming fresh foods and avoiding types that cause inflammation. The diet involves foods that are rich in oxidants, such as fresh fruits, vegetables, fatty fish, and beans. The foods you should avoid are mainly highly processed, deep-fried, and fast foods.

Anti-Inflammatory Diet and Calorie Count

Anti-inflammatory diets focus on balancing your daily macronutrient count between protein, fats, and carbohydrates. To follow an anti-inflammatory diet, you must consume 40 to 50 percent carbohydrates, 20 to 30 percent proteins, and 30 percent of fats daily. This is the distribution of the tota l calorie count. If you find it difficult tracking your calories, you can use calorie-tracking apps like MyFitnessPal, Life Sum, and Diet Coach.

Along with counting your daily calories, what's most important is sticking to anti-inflammatory foods. Eating rich anti-inflammatory foods and calorie counting are both compulsory for following this diet.

There is no gain if you maintain the recommended calorie count but incorporate processed and sugary foods into your diet. For instance, if you fulfill the 30 percent fat quota by eating a fried item, it is likely to cause inflammation instead of reducing it. Similarly, there is no benefit of loading up your plate with beneficial anti-inflammatory foods if it exceeds the macro-nutrient limit.

Guidelines for Anti-inflammatory Diet

Now that you have a good idea of what foods you need to consume, it is time to lay out some guidelines for following an anti-inflammatory diet.

Know the Healthy Carbohydrates

To incorporate healthy carbs in your diet, say goodbye to white starches and refined grains such as rice, white bread, pasta, and anything made with regular flour. Instead, opt for brown rice and whole grains. You can eat starchy vegetables like sweet potatoes and winter squash, so make sure to stock up on those as you can cook amazing and delicious recipes with them. Eat plenty of beans to fulfill your daily carbohydrate and protein count.

When limiting your carbohydrate intake on this diet, it is imperative to consume fiber-rich foods and drinks. Take at least 40 grams of fiber daily. A low carb diet, especially in the absence of fibers, can cause bowel problems such as constipation. The easiest way to fix your fiber intake is by eating berries, whole grains, cruciferous vegetables, and fruits.

Don't Miss on the Healthy Proteins

Where proteins-based foods are necessary for maintaining body functions, it is essential to differentiate between the healthy and not-so-healthy proteins. Your aim should be to eat more plant-based proteins and stay away from animal-based proteins such as chicken and beef. Instead, opt for fish and other seafood.

You can also enjoy beans, lentils, and soy, which are easy to make and beneficial for your body. Plant-based proteins are packed with essential amino acids, allowing them to fulfill your protein requirements while you avoid animal-based proteins.

If you want to enjoy the taste and texture of beef or chicken, go for tofu and tempeh. These plant-based proteins are a great alternative that tastes like meat and chicken. However, make sure you do not deep fry any of these healthy proteins.

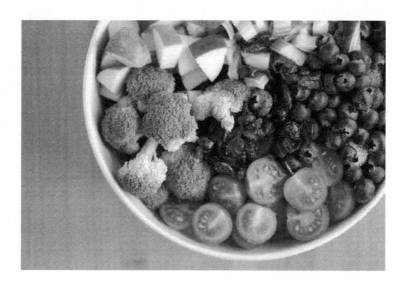

Enjoy Healthy Fats

When you are on an anti-inflammatory diet, it is necessary to consume more unsaturated fats and fewer saturated fats. Cook meals in olive oil, canola oil, avocado oil, grape seed or corn oil. Avoid butter and coconut oil and eat avocados, nuts, seeds, olives, and other plant-based healthy fats instead.

Say goodbye to trans-fats, which are found in processed foods and hydrogenated oil. Eat less full-fat dairy like butter, cheese, cream, and other dairy products — snack up on avocados, cashews, almonds, and walnuts. If you are concerned about GMOs, then go for organic canola oil.

Eating healthy fats means you can enjoy fatty fish. Eat sardines, mackerel, and salmon as they are rich in omega-3 fats and have sound anti-inflammatory effects. Other omega-3 rich foods include flax seeds and hemp seeds. Make your goal to eat fish at least twice a week.

Additional Guidelines

- Drink plenty of water. If you drink coffee or tea, make sure to drink it without any sugar.
- If you drink alcohol, choose red wine and drink in moderation.
- To satisfy your sweet tooth, delve on dark chocolate but in moderation.

Here is a table to summarize which foods you should and which foods you should not take.

Food groups	Anti-inflammation all-stars	Foods to avoid
Beans and legumes	✓	
Fruits	✓	
Allium vegetables	✓	
Cruciferous vegetables	✓	
Nightshade vegetables	✓	
Herbs and spices	✓	
Eggs	✓	
Fish	✓	
Red Meat		✓
White Meat		✓
White Bread, Rice Pastas		✓
Butter, Margarine		✓
Lard, Shortenings		✓
Nuts	✓	

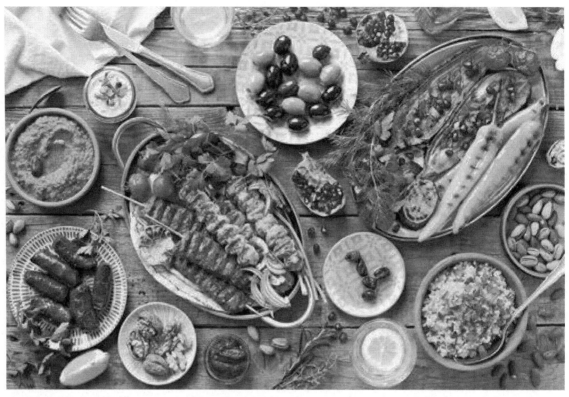

General Tips for Anti-Inflammatory Diet

- Include as much fresh food in your diet as possible. These include fresh fruits and vegetables.
- Avoid the consumption of processed foods as much as you can.
- Cut down on sugary beverages and sodas. You can have fresh fruit smoothies instead.
- Take extra care to stay within the daily calorie limit.
- Drink plenty of water.
- Maintain a proper sleeping routine.
- Exercise regularly to boost anti-inflammatory effects and metabolism.
- Add anti-inflammatory supplements such as omega-3 and turmeric in your foods.
- Carry anti-inflammatory snacks wherever you go to avoid purchasing fried and processed foods.
- Plan your shopping list ahead of time to ensure you are never out of healthy items and snacks for your anti-inflammatory diet.

Chapter 3: Ultimate Guide to Use a Slow Cooker

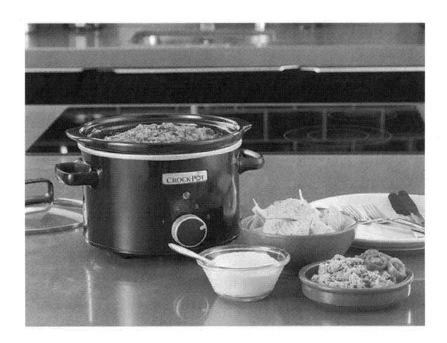

Following a strict diet plan is not easy. Not only you have to say goodbye to some of your favorite foods, but you also have to put in lots of time to prepare special meals that are not convenient for most people. Where following an anti-inflammatory diet can take most of your time for cutting ingredients, preparing seasonings, and cooking the food, a slow cooker comes as a savior reduces the amount of time you need to prepare delicious meals. All you need is one or two-step preparation and let the cooker do its work while you go about your routine work.

Slow Cooker is great for when you have to work long hours. Just add ingredients to the cooker before you leave, and when you come home, your meal is ready. That's right – it is safe for unattended cooking.

What is Slow Cooker, and How Does it Work?

A slow cooker or Crockpot is a design for a countertop electrical appliance. Being an electrical appliance, it is safe for unattended cooking since there is no danger of gas or fire involved. It is designed to cook foods at low or high temperatures for as long as 12 hours. It simmers the food at low temperatures rather than baking, frying, boiling and other cooking means that use high temperatures. Simmering foods at low temperature ensure that no nutrition of food is lost during cooking.

To understand how a slow cooker works, you need to get familiar with its parts. Slow cooker comprises three parts; the base, cooking vessel, and the lid.

The Base

The base allows you to hold and carry the vessel with a handle on its sides. It mostly contains a control knob or temperature panel to set the cooking temperature. At the bottom of the base, there are feet to keep the slow cooker above your countertop surface.

The base also contains a lining or heating band in the middle. The liner has thin metal inserted inside the construction of the slow cooker. You can't see or access the electrical workings of the liner inside the slow cooker. The heating bands or liner conducts the heat around the cooker to transfer it inside. The heat rises through the bottom and to the sides, cooking the food uniformly. There is a small amount of space between the liner and the outer material of the base. The small gap allows airflow so that the base does not overheat.

Cooking Vessel

The cooking vessel is usually made out of materials like heavy stoneware, which evenly distributes the heat, keeping it stable and constant inside. It is the portion where you put the food to be cooked.

How Does it Cook Food?

In terms of functioning, it is similar to a Ditch oven on the stovetop. A pot on a stovetop is heated from the bottom; the heat rises up to the sides and cooks the food within. Similarly, the base of the slow cooker creates heat and transfers it to the cooking vessel, effectively heating the food inside it. When you have to cook multiple things, add them to the bottom, where it takes the longest to cook.

When you set the temperature on the low setting to cook food, the heating element will put out less heat. On high temperatures, the heating band will create more heat. Cooking at low temperatures would obviously take more time than higher temperatures. The setting you choose depends upon the cooking time of the ingredients you will be using.

The Lid

The lid of the slow cooker is one of the main and very important components. It not only covers the food and avoids spills but is crucial to maintain the temperature for cooking. You probably won't be able to achieve an ideal cooking temperature without a lid. Imagine boiling pasta in the water with a lid on the pot and without a lid. The lid of the slow cooker works the very same way. Some slow cookers have a lid with clips to hold in place and provide convenience while traveling.

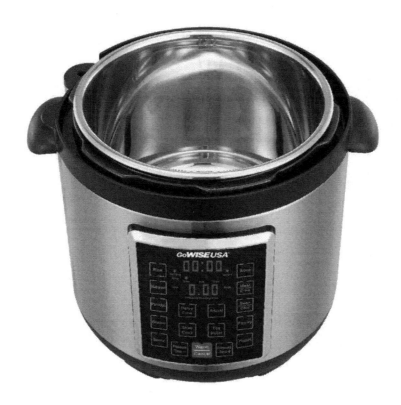

Understanding Slow Cooker Settings and Buttons

Slow cookers have two or three setting options for cooking food. For high temperatures, the food is likely to cook between 4 to 6 hours. On a low setting, the food cooks in 6 to 10 hours or even a little more. If possible, set the slow cooker on high setting in the first hour of the cooking and then adjust the setting according to your needs.

Note that one hour of the cooking time of high setting is equivalent to two hours of cooking on the low setting. One hour in the oven (350 degrees F) equals 4 hours on high and 8 hours on the low setting.

The buttons for settings are situated on the base. The number of buttons depends upon the slow cooker model you have. On some models, you'll find three separate buttons for the settings; off, low, and high. On others, you'll only find one - on these models, press the button until you get the desired setting, which you can view on the digital display. Follow the instruction manual to clean and use the slow cooker.

A thing to remember: If you are not going to be at home while the slow cooker is on, choose the 'warm' setting.

Slow Cooker Accessories

When you cook daily meals in the slow cooker, you will need certain accessories with it. You may not find all of these accessories essential, but trust me, they all are going to make your life much easier.

Oven Mitts

The slow cooker gets very hot after the cooking time. So, removing the pot without burning yourself can be tricky, especially if you're a beginner. A good pair of oven mitts is super convenient to remove the pot from a slow cooker and put on the table to serve the meal.

Slow Cooker Liners

If you find limited time to clean and maintain your slow cooker, then liners are perfect for you. Even if you do wash your slow cooker properly, it is good to have some liners at your disposal. The liner keeps your slow cooker clean when you have to make curries and similar dishes.

Though there are some pros and cons of using liners, make sure you get ones that are of good quality and are food grade. Using food-grade liners ensures there are no chemicals from the liners entering the food.

Microwavable Food Containers

Microwavable food containers are exactly not an accessory for a slow cooker, but they can be very handy. They are very useful for storing leftover food in the ridge, which you can reheat in the microwave. These containers are also great for taking meals to work or anywhere.

Slow Cooker Lid Lock

Not all slow cooker lids come with clippers. Lid lock kit has adjustable and flexible straps to hold the lid and can easily attach to the handle of the pot. With lid locks, lifting and moving a hot slow cooker is very easy.

Carry Bag

Keep a decent carry bag that can come in handy when you will need to carry your slow cooker. A good quality carry bag is insulated and keeps the crockpot, and the food inside, warm when traveling. You can find different sizes of carrying bags that fit your slow cooker.

Immersion Blender

Almost all the soups and stews recipes require an immersion blender to puree stuff. Without an immersion blender, it will take a lot of time to blend in batches separately. So, it is wise to have an immersion blender when you have to cook meals in a slow cooker.

Cooking Hacks for Slow Cooker

Now that you are well aware of how a slow cooker works, it's time to learn some cooking hacks that will make you love the slow cooker even more.

Two for One

Did you know you can make or reheat two dishes at a time in a slow cooker? Using a slow cooker liner allows you to reheat dips and soup at the same time. Place the liner in the slow cooker pot at the bottom and push it from between to make two cavities.

Double Boiler

A slow cooker can perfectly replace a double boiler. Simply fill it with a few inches of water and put whatever you need to melt in a glass or mason jar inside the cooker pot.

Catch Condensation

The slow cooker is great for making bread and brownies. However, the condensation can make them soggy at times. Use a warm cloth or a thick paper towel between the pot and lid to catch the drips of condensation, so they don't reach the food. Make sure the cloth or towel leaves no gap between the pot and lid.

Easily Remove Residue

With time, using a slow cooker can form a white residue layer, which is not easy to wash. Luckily, vinegar-baking soda hacks easily erase the white residue. Sprinkle baking soda on the pot and spray some vinegar. Leave for three to five minutes and wash off with warm soapy water.

Add Dairy Products Last

This is a very useful cooking hack for slow cookers. Milk and dairy products are emulsified blends of water and fats. Their texture can break apart when heated for a long period. To prevent this, add milk, cream, or cream cheese at the last minute before serving.

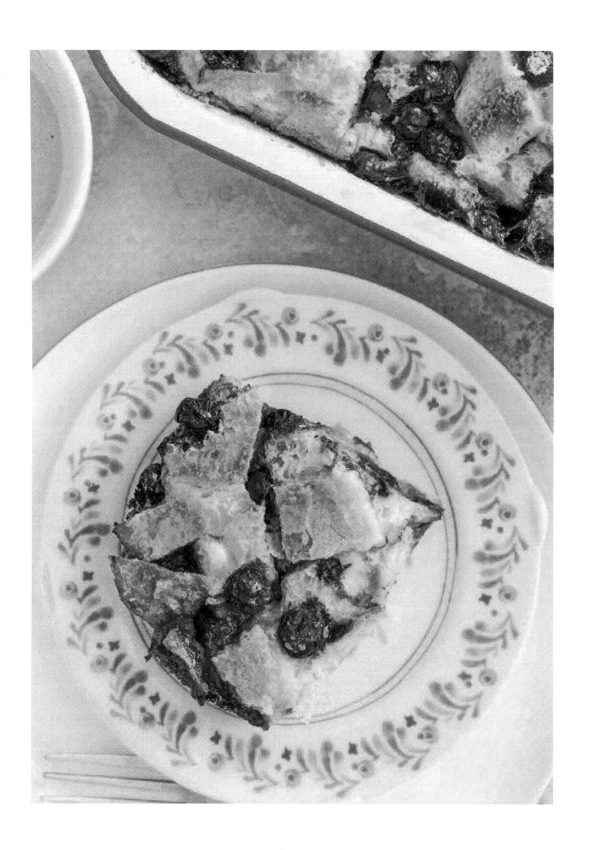

Chapter 4: 63 Amazing Anti-Inflammatory Slow Cooker Recipes

The most awaited part of the book is here. I am going to give you plentiful of mouth-watering and anti-inflammatory recipes that you can prepare in your slow cooker. Here, I have several categories of recipes to ensure that you have plenty of variety to choose from when on an anti-inflammatory diet.

Breakfast and Brunch

Before you go to sleep, prep your food in the slow cooker and have delicious anti-inflammatory meals for breakfast or brunch when you wake up.

Slow Cooker French toast Casserole

Prep time: 15 minutes, Cook time: 3-4 hours, Serves: 9

Ingredients:
- 2 eggs
- 2 egg whites
- 1 ½ almond milk or 1% milk
- 2 tbsp raw honey
- 1/2 tsp cinnamon
- 1 tsp vanilla extract
- 9 slices bread

For filling:
- 3 cups apples (diced)
- 2 tbsp raw honey
- 1 tbsp lemon juice
- 1/2 tsp cinnamon
- 1/3 cup of pecans

Instructions:
1. Add the first six ingredients into a bowl and mix.
2. Spray the insides of the slow cooker with a non-stick cooking spray.
3. Combine all the ingredients of the filling in a small bowl and set aside. Coat the apple pieces into the filling properly.
4. Cut slices of bread in half (triangle).
5. Place three slices on the bottom and some filing over. Layer the bread slices and filling in the same pattern.
6. Pour the egg mixture on top of the layers of bread and filling.
7. Set the cooker on high heat for 2 ½ hours or low heat for 4 hours.

Nutritional Facts per Slice:
Calories: 227, Total Fat: 7g, Saturated Fat: 1g, Carbohydrates: 34g, Protein: 9g, Sugar: 19g, Fiber 4g, Sodium: 187 mg, Cholesterol: 9mg

Crackpot Banana Foster

Prep time: 2 minutes, Cook time: 2 hours, Serves:

Ingredients:
- 1 tbsp melted coconut oil (unrefined)
- 3 tbsp honey
- 1/4 tsp cinnamon
- Juice of ½ medium-sized lemon
- 5 bananas (medium-sized)

For Garnish:
- Chopped nuts
- Greek Yogurt

Instructions:
1. Add the first four ingredients to the slow cooker and mix.
2. Cut the bananas in half and toss into the mixture inside the slow cooker.
3. Set on the cooker on low heat for 1 ½ to 2 hours.
4. Serve with chopped nuts or plain Greek yogurt.

Nutritional Facts per Serving:

Calories: 220, Total Fat: 4g, Saturated Fat: 2g, Carbohydrates: 56 g, Protein: 4g, Sugar: 36g, Fiber 4g, Sodium: 4 mg, Cholesterol: 0mg

Chicken and Quinoa Burrito Bowl

Prep time: 10 minutes, Cook time: 5 hours, Serves: 4-6

Ingredients:

- 1 lb. chicken thighs (skinless, boneless)
- 1 cup of chicken broth
- 1 can have diced tomatoes (14.5oz)
- 1 onion (chopped)
- 3 cloves garlic (chopped)
- 2 tsp chili powder
- ½ tsp coriander
- ½ tsp garlic powder
- 1 bell pepper (finely chopped)
- 15oz pinto beans (drained)
- 1 ½ cup cheddar cheese (grated)

Instructions:

1. Combine chicken, tomatoes, broth, onion, garlic, chili powder, garlic powder, coriander, and salt.
2. Set the cooker on low heat.
3. Remove the chicken from the cooker and shred into pieces with a fork and knife.
4. Put the chicken back in the slow cooker and add quinoa and pinto beans.
5. Set the cooker on low heat for 2 hours.
6. Add cheese on to the top and continue to cook and stir gently until the cheese melts.
7. Serve.

Nutritional Facts per 1/3 Serving Size:

Calories: 144mg, Total Fat: 39g, Saturated Fat: 19g, Carbohydrates: 68 g, Protein: 59g, Sugar: 8g, Fiber 17g, Sodium: 756 mg, Cholesterol: 144mg

Notes: You can substitute chicken thighs with chicken breasts, but thigh meat has denser texture and flavor. The chicken breast will taste a little dry in this recipe, so if you are using it, drizzle some olive oil over it.

Nutty Blueberry Banana Oatmeal

Prep time: 10 minutes, Cook time: 2-4 hours, Serves: 6

Ingredients:

- 2 cup rolled eats
- 1/4 cup almonds (toasted)
- 1/4 cup walnuts
- 1/4 cup pecans
- 2 tbsp ground flax seeds
- 1 tsp ground ginger
- 1 tsp cinnamon
- 1/4 tsp sea salt
- 2 tbsp coconut sugar
- ½ tsp baking powder
- 2 cups of milk
- 2 bananas
- 1 cup fresh blueberries
- 1 tbsp maple syrup
- 1 tsp vanilla extract or scraped vanilla bean
- 1 tbsp melted butter
- Yogurt for serving

Instructions:

1. In a large bowl, add nuts, flax seeds, baking powder, spices, and coconut sugar and mix.
2. In another bowl, beat eggs, milk, maple syrup, and vanilla extract.
3. Slice the bananas in half and layer them in the slow cooker pot with blueberries.
4. Add oats mixture and pour the milk mixture on the top.
5. Drizzle with melted butter,
6. Cook the slow cooker on low heat for 4 hours or on high heat for 4 hours. Cook till the liquid is absorbed oats are golden brown.
7. Serve warm and top it off with plain Greek yogurt.

Nutritional Facts per Serving Size:

Calories: 346 mg, Total Fat: 15g, Saturated Fat: 4g, Carbohydrates: 45g, Protein: 11g, Sugar: 17g, Fiber 7g, Sodium: 145 mg, Cholesterol: 39mg

Slow Cooker Steamed Cinnamon Apples

Prep time: 10 minutes, Cook time: 2-4 hours, Serves: 6

Ingredients:
- 8 apples (peeled, cored)
- 2 tsp lemon juice
- 2 tsp cinnamon
- ½ tsp nutmeg
- ¼ cup of coconut sugar

Instructions:
1. Add all the ingredients in the slow cooker pot.
2. Set the slow cooker pot on low setting for 3 to 4 hours or high setting for 2 to 2 ½ hours.
3. Cook till the apples are tender
4. Serve

Nutritional Facts per Serving Size:

Calories: 136 , Total Fat: 0g, Saturated Fat: 0g, Carbohydrates: 36g, Protein: 1g, Sugar: 26g, Fiber 5g, Sodium: 6mg, Cholesterol: 0mg

Carrot Rice with Scrambled Eggs

Prep time: 15 minutes, Cook time: 3 hours, Serves: 3

Ingredients:

For Sweet Tamari Soy Sauce
- 3 tbsp tamari sauce (gluten-free)
- 1 tbsp water
- 2-3 tbsp molasses

For Spicy Mix-ins
- 3 garlic cloves
- 1 small shallot (sliced)
- 2 long red chilies
- Pinch of ground ginger

For the Carrot Rice:
- 2 Tbsp sesame oil
- 5 eggs
- 4 large carrots
- 8 ounces sausage (chicken or any type of– gluten-free and minced).
- 1 tbsp sweet soy sauce
- 1 cup bean sprouts
- 1/2 cup fined diced broccoli
- salt and pepper to taste

For Garnish:
- Cilantro
- Asian chili sauce
- Sesame seeds

Instructions:

For the Sauce:
1. In saucepan boil molasses, water and tamari at a high flame.
2. Lower the flame after the sauce boils and cook till molasses is completely dissolved.
3. Place the sauce in a separate bowl.

For The Carrot Rice:
4. In a bowl, combine ginger, garlic onion, and red chilies.
5. To make rice out of the carrots, spiralize the carrots in a spiralizer.
6. Pulse the spiralized carrots in a food processor.
7. Cut broccoli into small dice like pieces

8. Add the sausage, carrots, broccoli, and the bean sprouts into the bowl of onion, ginger, garlic, and chilies.
9. Add the spicy mix of vegetables and the tamari sauce in the slow cooker pot.
10. Set the cooker on high heat for 3 hours or low heat for 6 hours.
11. Scramble two eggs in a non-stick frying pan or skillet.
12. Dish out the carrot rice and add scrambled eggs on top.
13. Garnish with sesame seeds, Asian chili sauce, and cilantro.

Notes: You can substitute red chili peppers with jalapenos or any peppers of your choice. The taste and spice level vary for different peppers, so the taste and spiciness of long red chili peppers compliments this recipe the best.

You can rice the carrots using a food processor if you don't have a spiralizer. But spiralizing the carrots before pulsing gives a firm texture and prevents the carrot rice from turning soggy afterward.

This recipe comparatively has a higher calorie count than most of the anti-inflammatory recipes here. So, if you have this dish for brunch, have a lighter meal or snack for dinner.

Nutritional Facts per 1/3 Serving Size:

Calories: 230 mg, Total Fat: 13.7g, Saturated Fat: 2.9g, Carbohydrates: 15.9g, Protein: 12.2g, Sugar: 8g, Fiber 4.4g, Sodium: 1060 mg, Cholesterol: 239mg.

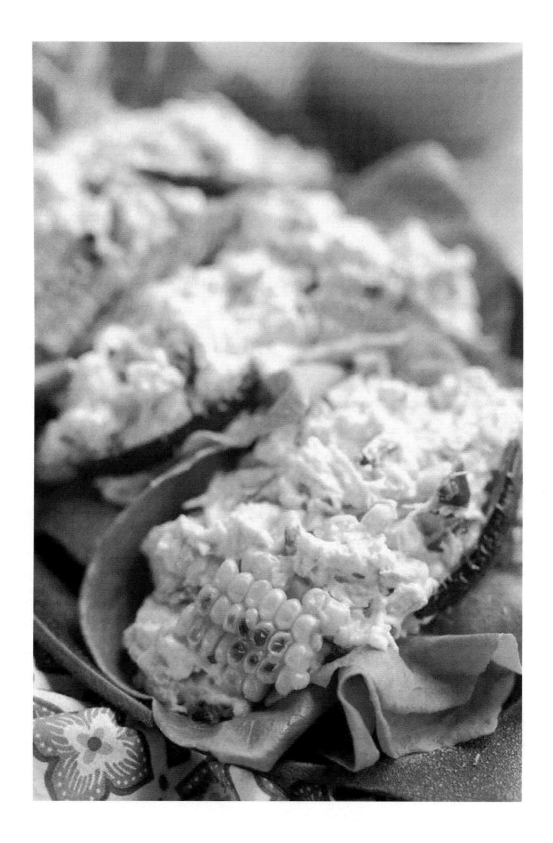

Salads

Eating salads every day can be boring. This is why we have included beef, chicken, and seafood slow cooker recipes in this book too. But when you are on an anti-inflammatory diet, it is better to include as many salads as you can in your meal plan. That's why we some very yummy and interesting anti-inflammatory salad recipe for you. Cooking salads in a slow cooker ensures that the flavors of seasonings and sauces are completely infused in the vegetables and proteins.

Slow Cooker Chicken Romaine Salad

This dish is fresh, flavorful, and, most importantly, it's anti-inflammatory! This super-duper chicken romaine salad can be enjoyed on its own or served with omelet, enchiladas, or sandwiches. The crunchy romaine lettuce leaves make a great healthy alternative for taco shells.

Prep time: 10 minutes, Cook time: 3 hours, Serves: 6

Ingredients:
- 3 tsp chili powder
- 1 tsp cumin
- 1 tsp salt
- 1 tsp pepper
- 1/2 tsp white pepper
- 1/2 tsp ground chipotle
- 1/2 tsp paprika
- 1/4tsp crushed red pepper flakes
- 1/4tsp dried oregano
- 1 ½ lb. chicken breast
- 1 cup chicken broth
- 9 cups torn romaine

For garnish (optional):
- sliced avocados
- chopped tomato
- sliced green onions

Instructions:
1. In a bowl, add all the seasonings and mix.
2. Rub the chicken breasts in the seasonings mix.
3. Add the seasoning and chicken breasts in the slow cooker pot.
4. Pour in the broth.
5. Cover the slow cooker and set it to cook for 3-4 hours on low heat or until the chicken is tender.
6. Take out the chicken and shred into pieces.
7. Place six romaine lettuce leaves on the serving platter.
8. Add shredded chicken to the romaine leaves.
9. Serve with thin avocado slices, chopped tomatoes, and green onions.

Nutritional Facts per Serving Size:
Calories:143, Total Fat: 3g, Saturated Fats: 1g, Carbohydrates: 4g, Protein: 24g, Sugar: 1g, Fiber: 2g, Sodium: 516mg, Cholesterol: 63mg

Slow-Cooked Kale with Smashed Garlic & Red Onions

Kale, Garlic, and Slow cooker? It is the perfect combination. This anti-inflammatory slow cooker salad preps in no time and gives you a complete meal. A sprig of rosemary and red onion slices gives a happy pop of color to this delicious kale salad.

Prep time: 10 minutes, Cook time: 2 hours, Serves: 6

Ingredients:
- 1/4 cup extra virgin olive oil
- 1 whole sprig rosemary
- 5-10 garlic cloves (smashed)
- 1 large red onion (sliced)
- 1/4 tsp red pepper flakes
- 1 lb. kale (center ribs removed)
- 1/2 tsp salt
- 1/2 tsp pepper

Instructions:
1. Remove the center ribs of the kale.
2. Cut the red onion in thin slices.
3. In a slow cooker pot, add garlic, red chili flakes, salt pepper, kale, rosemary, and onions.
4. Cover the pot and set it to cook on high heat for 2 hours or low heat for 4 hours.
5. Serve and Enjoy.

Nutritional Facts per Serving Size:

Calories: 202, Total Fat: 14.7g, Saturated Fats: 2.0g, Carbohydrates: 16g, Protein: 5.7g, Sugar: 4.2g, Fiber: 5.2g, Sodium: 46.3mg, Cholesterol: 119mg

Slow Cooker Avocado Chicken Salad

The star of this salad is avocado. Packed with different vitamins and anti-oxidants, this avocado chicken salad is not only healthy but has a fresh and creamy flavor that you can give add into your kid's sandwiches for school lunch too.

Prep time: 5 minutes, Cook time: 4 hours, Serves: 4-6

Ingredients:

- 1 1/2 lbs. chicken breasts
- 1 tbsp butter
- 2 garlic cloves (smashed)
- 2 sprigs thyme
- 1 tbsp parsley
- 1/4 onion (chopped)
- 1 ¼ cup chicken broth (low sodium)
- 1 cup of water
- 2 tbsp Dijon Mustard
- 2 tbsp parmesan cheese (grated)
- 1 tbsp lemon juice
- Salt pinch
- 1/2 tsp Pepper

Instructions:

1. Add chicken breasts, chicken, parsley, butter, smashed garlic, thyme, chicken broth, and water in the slow cooker. (To smash garlic, peel them and with the flat side of the knife smash the garlic while applying force with your palm.)
2. Cover the cooker pot and set it to cook on low heat for 4 hours.
3. Remove the chicken from the slow cooker pot after cooking.
4. Place the chicken into a large mixing bowl and shred with two forks.
5. Chop onions finely and add avocado slices, Dijon mustard, lemon juice, and parmesan cheese in a separate bowl and mix.
6. Add the mixture to the shredded chicken.
7. Mix the chicken and vegetables and toss evenly.
8. Add salt and pepper to taste and serve.

Notes: You can add green veggies and beans of your choice in this recipe.

Nutritional Facts per Serving Size:

Calories:211, Total Fat: 9g, Saturated Fats: 7g, Carbohydrates: 3.5g, Protein: 28g, Sugar: 0.2g, Fiber: 1g, Sodium: 240mg, Cholesterol: 119mg

Golden Tagine Crockpot Salad

This Moroccan-style tagine salad has warm sunny colors, making a perfect meal for winter nights. You can have it as a salad or a side dish.

Prep time: 10 minutes, Cook time: 4 hours, Serves: 6-8

Ingredients:

- 2 tbsp olive oil
- 1 medium-sized onion (chopped)
- 6 medium-sized carrots (diced)
- 2 cups butternut squash (cubed)
- 1lb rutabaga (1-inch chunks)
- 1 tbsp ginger (grated)
- 12 dried apricots
- 1 tsp cumin
- ½ tsp cinnamon
- ¼ tsp cayenne pepper
- ¼ tsp parsley or mint
- 2 cups chicken broth

Instructions:

1. Heat olive oil in a skillet over medium heat.
2. Sauté onions in the skillet.
3. Add onions, carrots, rutabaga, ginger, cumin, cinnamon, cayenne, butternut squash, apricots, and salt in a slow cooker pot. Pour the chicken broth on the top.
4. Cover and set the pot to cook for 4 hours on low heat.
5. Serve and sprinkle with parsley or mint leaves.

Nutritional Facts per Serving Size:

Calories:204, Total Fat: 11g, Saturated Fats: 4g, Carbohydrates: 27g, Protein: 31g, Sugar: 11g, Fiber: 7g, Sodium: 240mg, Cholesterol: 119mg

Slow Cooker Warm 3-Bean Salad

Low on fats, and high in fiber, this warm anti-inflammatory bean salad is a tasty and tangy way to boost your vegetable intake. With no sugar and a healthy amount of vinegar, this salad is tastier and tangier than your infamous canned salads.

Prep time: 10 minutes, Cook time: 4 hours, Serves: 10-12

Ingredients:
- ½ cup kidney beans (soaked overnight)
- ½ cup Canelli beans (soaked overnight)
- ¼ cup green beans
- ½ cup corn
- 1 can tomatoes(14 oz, diced)
- ¼ cup white vinegar
- 1 tsp pickling spice
- ½ tsp mustard seeds
- 1 cup of water
- hot pepper sauce to taste

Instructions:
1. In the slow cooker, add all the beans, green beans, corn, tomatoes, vinegar, pickling spice, and mustard seeds.
2. Pour water on the top.
3. Cover the pot and set to cook for 4 hours on low heat.
4. Serve warm with some hot sauce.

Notes: The spiciness of pepper intensifies during slow cooking so if you want the salad to be less spicy, then add half the amount of spice.

Nutritional Facts per Serving Size:

Calories:100, Total Fat: 0.5g, Saturated Fats: 0.0g, Carbohydrates: 19.4g, Protein: 6g, Sugar: 2g, Fiber: 5g,

Curtido Cabbage Salad

This cabbage salad is actually a healthier, chunkier, and yummier version of coleslaw. Prepared in the slow cooker, this curtido cabbage salad can be eaten on its own or as a side dish. Kids will love it in their sandwich.

Prep time: 15 minutes, Cook time: 3 hours, Serves: 10

Ingredients:

- 2 cups green cabbage (shredded)
- 2 cups red cabbage (shredded)
- 1 medium red pepper
- 1 cup onion (thin rings)
- 3 carrots (diced)
- 1 cup green beans (1-inch pieces)
- 1/2tsp dried oregano
- 1/2cup zesty Italian dressing
- 1/4cup vinegar
- ½ tsp salt

Instructions:

1. In a bowl, add zesty Italian dressing, vinegar, salt, and oregano and mix.
2. Add green cabbage, red cabbage, green beans, onion, carrots, and red pepper(cut in wide strips) into the bowl.
3. Toss the vegetables well in the Italian dressing mixture.
4. Transfer into the slow cooker pot.
5. Cover the pot and set it to cook for 3 hours on low heat or 1 1/2 hours on high heat.
6. Let it cool and refrigerate an hour before serving.

Nutritional Facts per Serving Size:

Calories: 60, Total Fat: 3g, Saturated Fats: 0g, Carbohydrates: 7g, Protein: 18g, Sugar: 4g, Fiber: 2g, Sodium: 440mg, Cholesterol: 0mg

Slow Cooker Hot German Potato Salad

This amazing dish is ideal for lunch, dinner, and parties. The addition of bacon imparts flavor and texture to this salad, complementing the sweet potatoes.

Prep time: 15 minutes, Cook time: 5 hours, Serves: 12

Ingredients:

- 1 ¼ cup bacon (chopped)
- 3 medium onions (chopped)
- 5 medium celery stalks(chopped)
- 1 lb. small red potatoes
- 2 tsp pepper
- ¾ tsp celery seed
- 1 1/2 tsp salt
- 1 cup chicken broth
- ¼ cup sugar
- 2 tbsp corn starch
- ¼ cup cider vinegar
- 2 tbsp parsley (chopped)

Instructions:

1. In a 12-inch skillet, cook bacon over medium heat. Stir frequently until crisp and brown.
2. Remove bacon from the skillet and drain on paper towels using a slotted spoon.
3. Cook celery and onion in the bacon dripping in the skillet for 5 to 8 minutes. Stir frequently and cook until the onion and celery are tender and crisp.
4. Season with salt, pepper, and celery seed and refrigerate.
5. Cut sweet potatoes in ¼-inch slices about 2-3 inches in diameter.
6. Place a few slices of sweet potatoes in the slow cooker pot. Layer with bacon mix and repeat the layering.
7. Pour the broth on top. Cover and cook for 5-6 hours on low heat.
8. Remove potatoes from the cooker with a slotted spoon. In a small bowl, mix vinegar, sugar, and cornstarch.
9. Fold the potatoes in the liquid and transfer back in the slow cooker pot.
10. Cover and cook for another 20-30 minutes on high heat or until the potatoes have thickened.
11. Serve hot.

Notes: You can omit the bacon if you want to or replace it with chicken, beef, or tofu strips.

Nutritional Facts per Serving Size:

Calories: 130, Total Fat: 3g, Saturated Fats: 1g, Carbohydrates: 22g, Protein: 18g, Sugar: 7g, Fiber: 3g, Sodium: 480mg, Cholesterol: 0mg

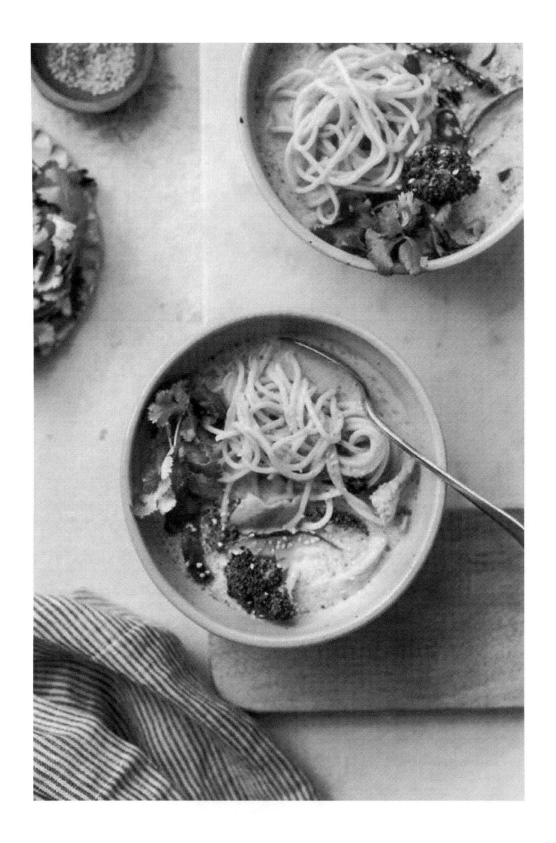

Soups and Stews

Healthy Broccoli Curry Soup

Prep time: 15 minutes, Cook time: 7 hours; Serves 5

Ingredients:

- 1 lb. Organic Chicken Breasts (Boneless and Skinless, 4 oz chopped pieces)
- 6 stalks Celery (chopped into about one-inch pieces)
- 5 Carrots (chopped into one-inch pieces)
- 1/2 Red Onion (one-inch tall pieces)
- 2 cups of Broccoli (florets)
- 2 cups of Cauliflower (florets)
- 2 tsp or 4 cloves of Minced Garlic
- 32 oz Low Sodium Chicken Broth (Organic)

Seasoning:

- 1 tsp Garlic Powder
- 3/4 tsp Basil
- 1 tsp Curry Powder
- 1/2 tsp Cumin Powder
- 1 tsp Paprika
- 1/4 tsp Turmeric
- 1/2 tsp Onion Powder
- 1/4 tsp Black Pepper

Instructions:

1. Chop the vegetables and chicken accordingly.
2. Combine all the seasonings in a separate bowl and mix.
3. In a slow cooker pot, add ingredients in the following order: Chicken on the bottom, carrots, celery, onions, broccoli, cauliflower, minced garlic, seasoning.
4. Pour the chicken broth on top of it all (Make sure to add everything in the right order as some things cook faster than others.)
5. Press the 'cook' button and adjust the cooking time for seven hours on regular heat. You will probably need to adjust the cooking time for this recipe if you are using a regular slow cooker. (I use low heat for 7 1/2 to 8 hours)

Nutrition Facts Per Serving:

Calories: 180, Fat: 3.1g, Saturated Fat: 0.8g, Carbohydrates: 14.9g, Protein: 24.7g, Sugar: 6.1g, Fiber: 5g, Sodium: 275mg, Cholesterol: 52mg

Best Detox Lentil Soup

Prep time: 1/2 hour, Cook time: 6 hours; Serves 8

Ingredients:

For Slow cooker:
- 2 cups carrots (sliced)
- 2 cups butternut squash (cubes)
- 2 cups celery
- 2 cups potato
- 1 onion
- 1 cup green lentils
- 3/4 cup yellow split peas
- 5 cloves garlic (minced)
- 8-10 cups chicken or vegetable broth
- 2 tsp herb de Provence
- 1 tsp salt

For Garnish:
- 2 cups kale (roughly chopped)
- 1 cup parsley (chopped)
- ½ cup olive oil or rosemary oil
- few drops of lemon juice

Instructions:

1. Place all the slow cooker ingredients and cook on high setting for 5-6 hours or 7-8 hours for a low setting.
2. In a blender, add 4 cups of soup with olive or rosemary oil. Pulse gently until the soup has a creamy consistency.
3. Add the soup into the pot again and combine kale and parsley. Add a swish of lemon for a little tanginess.
4. Allow the soup to cool down a bit before serving. It improves the taste and texture.

Nutrition Facts per Serving:

Calories: 322, Fat: 14.8g, Carbohydrates: 39.5g, Protein: 10.8g, Fiber:13.2g, Sodium: 906.3mg, Cholesterol: 0mg

Broccoli Turmeric Soup

Prep time: 10 minutes, Cook time: 4-8 hours, Serves 4

Ingredients:
- 2 cups of leek or yellow onions (chopped)
- 1 cup carrot (diced)
- 2 tbsp fresh ginger (chopped)
- 4 cups of broccoli (small florets)
- 1 tsp turmeric
- ¼ tsp red pepper (crushed)
- ½ tsp ground cumin
- 2 cloves garlic (minced)
- 3 cups of vegetable broth

Instructions:
1. Combine all ingredients in your slow cooker.
2. Set the cooker on high heat for 4 hours or low heat for 8 hours.
3. Use an immersion blender to puree the soup. Serve hot.

Nutrition Facts per Serving:

Calories: 77g, Total Fat: 1g, Saturated Fats: 0g, Carbohydrates: 16 g, Protein: 4g, Sugar: 5g, Fiber 4g, Sodium: 318 gm, Cholesterol: 0g

Seafood Ste

Prep time: 15 minutes, Cook time: 3hours and 30 minutes, Serves 6

Ingredients:

- 1 can crushed tomatoes (28oz)
- 1 tbsp tomato puree
- 3 cloves garlic (minced)
- 4 cups of vegetable broth
- 1 cup of onion (cubed)
- 1 large or 2 medium-sized potatoes (small pieces)
- 1 tbsp dried basil
- 1 tsp dried thyme
- 1/4 tsp crushed red pepper
- 1/8 tsp cayenne pepper
- 1/2 tsp salt
- 1/2 tsp black pepper
- 1 tsp oregano
- 2 pounds seafood of choice (Suggested: 1 pound large shrimp and 1 pound scallops)
- A handful of parsley (chopped)

Instructions:

1. Add all the ingredients, except for the seafood, in your slow cooker. Cover the pot and cook on high setting for 2-3 hours or low setting for 4-6 hours. The potatoes should be properly cooked through.
2. Add thawed seafood in the slow cooker. Turn on high heat and cook for 30-60 minutes until the seafood is cooked
3. Garnish the stew with chopped parsley, Serve with crusty bread.

Nutrition Facts per Serving

Calories: 111, Total Fat: 1g, Saturated Fats: 0g, Carbohydrates: 19 g, Protein: 6g, Sugar: 5g, Fiber 4g, Sodium: 1338 gm,

Slow Cooker Peasant Stew

Prep time: 15 minutes, Cook time: 3-4 hours, Serves 6

Ingredients:
- 6 boneless chicken thighs (skinless preferred)
- 2 tsp olive oil
- 1 large onion (chopped)
- 1 tsp ground cumin
- Salt and pepper
- 16 oz can of kidney beans (rinsed and drained)
- 16 oz can of pinto beans
- 10 oz can have diced tomatoes (un-drained)
- 1/2 cup of fresh parsley (chopped)
- 1-2 tbsp sour cream

Instructions:
1. Rub chicken thighs with salt, pepper, and cumin.
2. In a skillet, add olive oil on medium heat. Cook chicken thighs for five minutes or until both sides turn brown.
3. Add canned tomatoes in the slow cooker.
4. Add onions in the cooker and place cooked chicken on top.
5. Cook the stew for 3 to 4 hours. Puree with an immersion blender after the soup is cooked.
6. Add beans and cook for another hour.
7. Garnish with cilantro and sour cream. Serve hot.

Nutrition Facts per Serving

Calories: 463, Total Fat: 2g, Saturated Fats: 0g, Carbohydrates: 20.1g, Protein: 28.9g, Sugar: 5.3g, Fiber 4.1g, Sodium: 407 gm,

Healthy Chicken Pot Pie Stew

Prep time: 5 minutes, Cook time: 4 hours, serves: 6

Ingredients:

- 1 lb. chicken breasts (boneless and skinless)
- 1 large onion (diced)
- 3 carrots (diced)
- 3 stalks celery (diced)
- 3 garlic cloves (minced)
- 1 ½ tsp kosher salt
- 1 tsp oregano
- 1 tsp dried thyme
- 1bay leaf
- 1 tsp black pepper
- 3 ½ cups of chicken broth

For garnish:

- 1/3 cup peas
- 1/3 cup frozen pearl onions
- 1/3 cup frozen corn kernel
- 1/2 cup of Greek yogurt

Instructions:

1. Combine chicken breasts, onions, carrots, celery, garlic, all the spices, and chicken broth in the slow cooker pot. Stir all the things.
2. Add in a bay leaf and cover the pot.
3. Cook on low heat for 4-5 hours. Make sure the chicken is cooked and vegetables are tender in the end.
4. Remove the bay leaf.
5. Take out the chicken breasts and shred. Keep the shredded chicken aside.
6. Puree the soup with an immersion blender or use a blending machine to blend the soup in batches.
7. Add the shredded chicken back to the slow cooker. Combine frozen vegetables and Greek yogurt.
8. Cover the slow cooker pot and cook for another 30 minutes until the vegetables are heated enough.
9. Season with salt and pepper. Serve hot.

Nutrition Facts per Serving:

Calories: 314, Total Fat: 9.1g, Saturated Fats: 2.7g, Carbohydrates: 17.3 g, Protein: 38.4g, Sugar: 7.3g, Fiber 3.5g, Sodium: 225 gm

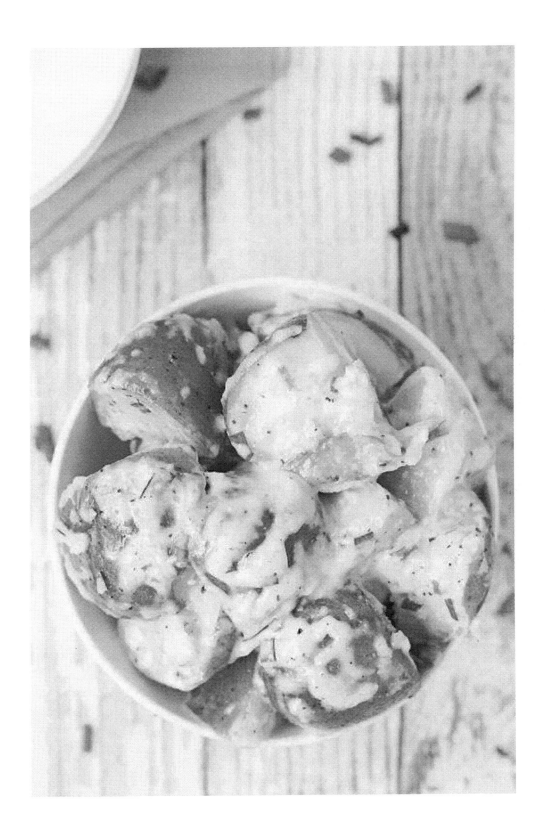

Appetizers and Snacks

Here are the best anti-inflammatory and healthy recipes for appetizers and snacks. They are easy to make and take to work when you have to satisfy your untimely hunger pangs.

Crockpot Baked Sweet Potatoes

Prep time: 3 minutes, Cook time: 5-7hours, Serves: 6

Ingredients:
- 2 tsp olive oil
- 3 large sweet potatoes
- For Garnish (optional):
- Dried Fruit
- Thin slivers of ginger
- Plain Greek Yoghurt

Instructions:
1. Brush the sweet potatoes with some olive oil.
2. Cover the potatoes with food-grade foil and put in the slow cooker for 5-7 hours on low setting or until the sweet potatoes are tender enough.
3. Take out the potatoes carefully with tongs as they will be too hot.
4. Remove the foil from each potato and cut in into thick slices.
5. Garnish with plain Greek yogurt. You can top it off with either dried fruits or thinly sliced ginger.

Notes: Some people have asked me about not adding the water, so there is no need. The steam of the slow cooker can perfectly cook the sweet potatoes without any water.

Nutritional Facts per Serving:

Calories: 142, Total Fat: 0g, Carbohydrates: 32 g, Protein: 4g, Sugar: 1g, Fiber 4g, Sodium: 11 mg, Cholesterol: 0mg

Slow-Cooked Salsa

Prep time: 15 minutes, Cook time: 2 ½ hours, Serves: 2

Ingredients:
- 10 plum tomatoes
- 2 garlic cloves
- 1 small onion, cut into wedges
- 2 jalapeno peppers
- 1/4 cup cilantro leaves
- 1/2 teaspoon salt, optional

Instructions:
1. Core the tomatoes. Cut a slit in between the tomatoes and insert a garlic clove into each slit.
2. Add tomatoes and onions in the slow cooker pot.
3. Cut stems off the jalapenos and add them into the slow cooker pot.
4. Cover the pot and set it on high heat for 2 ½ -3 hours until the vegetables are properly cooked.
5. After the cooking time, blend the vegetables with an immersion blender to form a tomato salsa.
6. Season with salt and cilantro.
7. You can enjoy the salsa with homemade or gluten-free nachos.

Caution: Wear gloves when cutting the hot jalapenos. The oils in the jalapeno can burn your skin. Be careful and do not touch your face or skin without washing your hands.

Nutritional Facts per Serving:

Calories: 80, Total Fat: 0g, Carbohydrates: 16 g, Protein: 4g, Sugar: 12g, Fiber 4g, Sodium: 20mg, Cholesterol: 0mg

Crockpot Ginger Bread Latte

Prep time: 5 minutes, Cook time: 5 hours, serves: 8

Ingredients:
- 6 cups of skim milk
- 2 tbsp coconut sugar
- 4 tbsp maple syrup
- 3 tsp ground ginger
- 2 cinnamon sticks
- 1 tsp vanilla extract
- 1/2 tsp ground nutmeg
- 3 cups of strong brewed coffee

Instructions:
1. Add all the ingredients into the slow cooker and cover. Put the cooker on low setting for 3 hours.
2. Stir the pot occasionally.
3. Set the slow cooker on 'keep warm' setting and cook for another two hours.
4. Stir the mixture making sure that it does not boil.
5. Pour into the serving cups and enjoy.

Notes: If you want to enjoy anti-inflammatory pumpkin spice latte, then use the same recipe and add a can of pumpkin puree instead of ginger. You can even make a combination of pumpkin and ginger latte by adding a teaspoon of ground ginger with the pumpkin puree.

Nutritional Facts per Serving:

Calories: 109, Total Fat: 0g, Carbohydrates: 20 g, Protein: 7g, Sugar: 18g, Fiber 0g, Sodium: 101 mg, Cholesterol: 0mg

Anti-Inflammatory Cauliflower Fried Rice

Prep time: 40 minutes, Cook time: 3-4 hours, Serves: 8

Ingredients:
- 2 cauliflower (heads)
- 2 tbsp ginger garlic paste
- 2 eggs
- 1/2 cup of vegetable broth
- 1 cup of mix frozen veggies
- 1/2 cup of diced turkey (optional)

For Garnish:
- 1/2 cup cilantro (chopped)
- 1/2 cup green onions (chopped)
- 2tsp low sodium soy sauce

Instructions:
1. Cut the cauliflower head into florets and discard the stems.
2. Put the florets into a food processor. Pulse the cauliflower florets to form fine crumbs.
3. Add the cauliflower crumbs, ginger-garlic paste, and vegetable broth into the slow cooker.
4. Cover the pot and cook on low setting for 3-4 hours or 2-2 ½ hours on high setting.
5. Whisk the eggs and make scrambled eggs in a skillet.
6. When the cauliflower mix is cooked, add eggs, frozen veggies, and diced turkey. Cook for another 30 minutes on the low heat.
7. Add seasonings: Green onions, cilantro, and soya sauce for taste.

Nutritional Facts per Serving:
Calories: 86, Total Fat: 2g, Saturated Fat: 1g, Carbohydrates: 11 g, Protein: 7g, Sugar: 3g, Fiber 4g, Sodium: 201 mg, Cholesterol: 46mg

Notes: You can sue the same recipe as a full meal for lunch or dinner. For a full meal, this recipe serves a large portion per person, serving 4 instead of 8.

Cranberry Poached Pears

Prep time: 10 minutes, Cook time: 3-4 hours, Serves: 6

Ingredients:

- 6 pears (peeled)
- 6 cups of fresh or unsweetened canned cranberry juice
- ¼ coconut palm sugar
- Peels of one orange
- 1 cup of raisins
- 3 sticks of cinnamon
- 1 tsp ground ginger or ginger powder
- 2 pods of star anise (optional)
- 3 tbsp arrowroot starch

For Garnish:

- 6-8 mint leaves (optional)
- Plain Greek Yogurt

Instructions:

1. In a slow cooker pot, combine cranberry juice, orange peel, cinnamon sticks, raisins, star anise, and ground ginger. Add pears into the pot.
2. Cook the pears in the cranberry juice for 3-4 hours on the low heat setting. The pears will float in the juice, so keep stirring occasionally.
3. Take half a cup of the poaching liquid from the slow cooker into the bowl. Whisk arrowroot into the poaching liquid.
4. Strain the slow cooker pot to remove the ginger, cinnamon, star anise, and raisins. Save the raisins for garnishing.
5. Heat the pot again on high setting and add the arrowroot mixture.
6. When the mixture boils, reduce the heat and cook for another 5 minutes till there is a syrup-like consistency.
7. Take out the pears and let them cool for a bit.
8. Pour the cranberry syrup over the poached pears.
9. Garnish with raisins and a dollop of yogurt. Add in some mint leaves if you want to.

Notes: You can substitute coconut palm sugar with pure raw honey or pure agave nectar. If you do not have arrowroot starch, you can use 2 tablespoons of cornstarch instead.

Nutritional Facts per Pear:

Calories: 224, Total Fat: 0g, Saturated Fat: 0g, Carbohydrates: 58 g, Protein: 1g, Sugar: 46g, Fiber 46g, Sodium: 8 mg, Cholesterol: 0mg

Slow Cooker Cheddar Polenta with Winter Greens

Prep time: 5 minutes, Cook time: 2 hours, Serves: 4

Ingredients:

Polenta:
- 2 cups of milk
- 2 tbsp butter
- 1/3 cup cornmeal or corn grits
- 1/4 cup half and a half (low fat cream and milk)
- 3/4 cup grated cheddar cheese

Greens:
- 2 tbsp olive oil
- 3 cloves garlic (minced)
- 1lb dark leafy winter greens (collards, lake, chard, etc.)
- 1 tbsp fresh lemon juice
- Sea salt and pepper to taste

Instructions:
1. To make the polenta, add cornmeal or corn grits with milk into a saucepan.
2. Bring it to boil and stir in softened or melted butter. Add salt and pepper to taste.
3. Transfer the polenta into the slow cooker and set on the low heat for 2 hours.
4. To prepare the greens, begin with heating a large skillet over medium heat. Add olive oil and minced garlic and sauté for a minute.
5. Add leafy winter greens and cook in the skillet for two to three minutes until the veggies are wilted. Add lemon juice over the green veggies.
6. Add half and half, and cheddar cheese into the polenta. Then, stir.
7. Scoop out the polenta into the serving bowls and top with green beans. Enjoy warm and yummy polenta with healthy winter greens.

Nutritional Facts per Serving:

Calories: 473, Total Fat: 22g, Saturated Fat: 10g, Carbohydrates: 52 g, Protein: 19g, Sugar: 7g, Fiber 8g, Sodium: 273 mg, Cholesterol: 45mg

Notes: This recipe has a good amount of dairy. Make sure you do not eat other meals that have dairy when you are having cheddar polenta and green beans for appetizer or lunch.

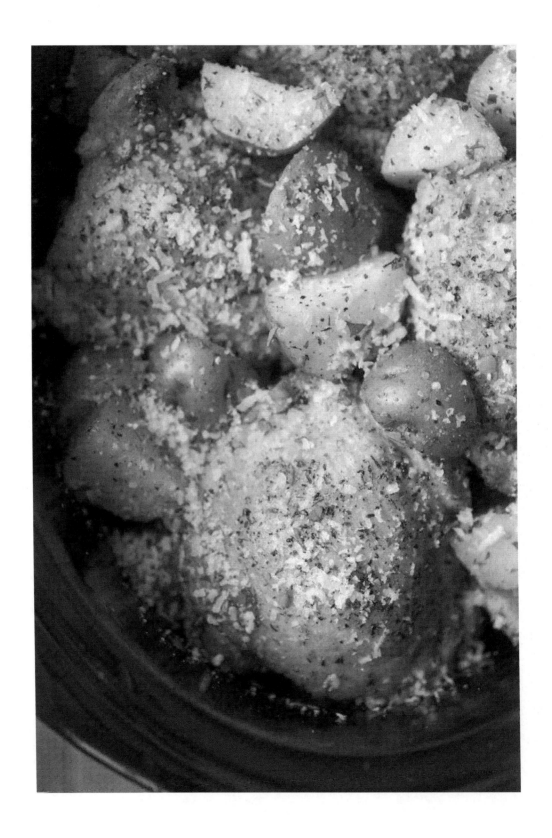

Vegetables and Vegan

Here is the most important recipe section of this book. Yes, I am talking about the vegetables. By now, you must know that plant-based foods mainly are anti-inflammatory. Most vegetables are rich in antioxidants and other compounds that help fight off inflammation. Although we have listed a variety of anti-inflammatory recipes in this book, do not miss out on including these vegetable and vegan recipes in your anti-inflammatory diet.

Slow Cooker Vegan Gumbo

If you love Southern food, then you will love this vegan gumbo too. The flavors are bold and spicy, loaded with the goodness of gumbo beans. Sothern gumbo beans traditionally use meat, chicken, or sausage in combination. But this hearty bowl of gumbo has kidney beans and mushrooms instead to make the beans filling and delicious for you. You can enjoy this dish with brown rice.

Prep time: 10 minutes, Cook time: 8 hours, Serves: 10

Ingredients:
- 1 onion (chopped)
- 1 green bell pepper (chopped)
- 2 stalks celery (chopped)
- 2 large carrots (chopped)
- 2 can tomatoes (15 oz)
- 1 ½ cup asparagus or okra
- 1 ½ cup mushrooms
- 1 cup kidney beans
- 2 tbsp soy sauce
- 2 tbsp Cajun seasoning
- 1/2 tsp salt
- 1/2 tsp dried thyme
- 2 tbsp tomato paste
- 1/4 cup parsley (chopped)

Instructions:
1. Soak kidney beans in water overnight or at least for 6 hours before cooking.
2. In a slow cooker, add gumbo beans, kidney beans, mushrooms, bell peppers, onions, celery, carrots, diced tomatoes, soy sauce, Cajun seasoning, salt, and thyme.
3. Mix well and cover the pot. Set the pot to cook on low heat for 8 hours or high heat for 4 hours.
4. Add tomato paste and cook for another 30 minutes for 20-30 minutes or until thickened.
5. Garnish with chopped parsley and serve with brown rice.

Notes: For gumbo beans, you can use asparagus, okra, or a mix of both.

Nutritional Facts per Serving Size:
Calories: 261, Total Fat: 2g, Saturated Fats: 0g, Carbohydrates: 51g, Protein: 13g, Sugar: 10g, Fiber: 13g, Sodium: 892mg, Cholesterol: 0mg

Slow Cooker Loaded Baked Potato Casserole

If you think all the recipes in this section are going to be about leafy greens and slow-cooked vegetables, then here is a treat for you. This recipe is your ultimate comfort food fix for days when you will feel bored with eating all the vegetables.

As this casserole has yogurt and cream cheese in it, I have included a vegan cream cheese version in this recipe, just to limit the amount of dairy. If you are not strictly vegan, you can use good old plain Greek yogurt or else substitute it with non-dairy vegan yogurt.

Prep time: 15 minutes, Cook time: 4 hours, Serves: 6

Ingredients:

- 3 pounds potatoes (skin on)
- 1 cup vegetable broth (low sodium)
- 1/2 cup Greek yogurt (fat-free)
- 1/2 cup vegan cream cheese
- 1/2 cup tofu cooked (optional)
- 1/2 tsp black pepper
- 1/4 cup green onion

For Vegan Cream Cheese:

- 1 ¼ cup raw cashew or macadamia nuts
- 1/4 cup non-dairy yogurt or water
- 1 ½ tbsp cider vinegar
- Salt to taste

Instructions:

1. Cut the potatoes in quarter pieces and place them in the slow cooker.
2. Pour the vegetable broth on the potatoes and cook for 4 hours on high heat. Add more water if the broth gets completely absorbed.
3. Meanwhile, for the cream cheese, soak the cashews or macadamia nuts for 2-3 hours in water.
4. Drain the water and blend nuts, with non-dairy yogurt or water, salt, and vinegar in a food processor.
5. Your vegan cream cheese is ready
6. Coming back to the casserole, Mash the potatoes when tender. Do not drain the water.
7. Add in the yogurt, vegan cream cheese, tofu, pepper, and sliced green onions and mix well.
8. Cover the slow cooker and let it sit for 5-10 minutes.
9. Serve and enjoy.

Nutritional Facts per Serving Size (about ½ cup):

Calories: 332, Total Fat: 12g, Saturated Fats: 6g, Carbohydrates: 43g, Protein: 15g, Sugar: 4g, Fiber: 5g, Sodium: 305mg, Cholesterol: 30mg

Slow Cooker Stuffed Bell Pepper

Bell peppers are great to add crunch to salads and wraps. But, they also make a wonderful dish when left unsliced. Hollow bell peppers are ideal for adding stuffing, making an awesome alternative to wraps and other carbs. When cooked in the crockpot, bell peppers become soft and flavorful. These stuffed bell peppers are great for weekend dinner.

For this stuffed bell pepper recipe, beans and tomatoes make a healthy and amazing stuffing. This recipe also calls for cheese to top on the stuffing, but you can omit the cheese if you want to, they will still taste great.

Prep time: 20 minutes, Cook time: 4hours, Serves: 5

Ingredients:
- 2 tsp olive oil
- 1 medium onion (diced)
- 4 cloves garlic (minced)
- 2 ribs celery (diced)
- 2 tsp ground cumin
- 1 tbsp chili powder
- 1 ½ tsp oregano
- 1 ½ cup black beans
- 1 ½ cup pinto beans
- 1 cup corn kernels
- 1 large tomato (diced)
- 1 canned chipotle pepper in adobo (minced)
- Salt to taste
- 5 large bell peppers
- 1/2 cup enchilada sauce
- ¼ cup shredded pepper jack (optional)

Instructions:
1. Soak black beans and pinto beans separately in water overnight.
2. In a large skillet, heat olive oil over medium heat. Add onion and celery cook until brown for about 5 minutes. Stir often while cooking.
3. In a large bowl, combine garlic, chili powder, oregano, cooked onion, celery, drained beans, tomatoes and corn, and mix well.
4. Add salt and pepper to taste and mix.
5. Next, cut the tops of bell peppers and remove the seeds and pith.
6. Spoon the stuffing into bell peppers. If you wish to add cheese, then fill half of the pepper with stuffing. Do not add the cheese yet.
7. Place the bell peppers in the slow cooker. Fill water that covers at least half of the peppers, around two cups. Be careful when pouring water; make sure water does not get into the pepper.
8. Cover the slow cooker pot and cook for 3 ½ - 4 hours on low heat, until they can be easily pierced with a fork but still hold their shape.
9. Add cheese in the last fifteen minutes of the cooking and cook till the cheese is melted.
10. Carefully remove the hot peppers with the help of tongs. Spoon one to two tablespoons of enchilada sauce on top of the bell peppers and serve.

Slow Cooker Eggplant Lasagna

Who doesn't love lasagna? I am sure you do too. Here is a recipe, which, after eating, you won't mind becoming a vegetarian. This vegetarian version of lasagna is anti-inflammatory, nutrient-rich, and yummy.

Instead of noodles, the lasagna comprises delicious eggplant layers. Made with loads of veggies, sugar-free tomato sauce, and low-fat cheese, this recipe is sure to make you feel healthy and awesome.

Prep time: 15 minutes, Cook time: 3 hours, Serves: 6

Ingredients:
- 2 eggplants
- 1 egg
- 1 cup cottage cheese (low-fat)
- 1 cup mozzarella cheese (low-fat)
- 1 jar sugar-free spaghetti sauce (24oz)
- 1 tsp salt
- 1 onion (diced)
- 1 bell pepper (diced)

Instructions:
1. Peel the eggplants and cut into thin slices that resemble lasagna noodle sheets.
2. Lay the eggplant slices on a power towel and sprinkle with salt and pepper. Let sit for 10-15 for excess moisture to drain.
3. In the meantime, combine cottage cheese, mozzarella, and egg in a mixing bowl.
4. Add 1/4cup of tomato sauce in the slow cooker pot: layer eggplant slices, peppers, onions, egg, and cheese mix. Repeat the layers three times or as per your requirement.
5. Cover the pot and cook for 5-6 hours on low heat or 3-4 hours on high heat.

Nutritional Facts per Serving Size:
Calories: 211, Total Fat: 10g, Saturated Fats: 5g, Carbohydrates: 719g, Protein: 14g, Sugar: 10g, Fiber: 3g, Sodium: 802mg, Cholesterol: 58mg

Slow Cooker Ratatouille

Since the movie came out, Ratatouille has been a very popular dish among the chef and home cooks. It is a fancy dish that uses no fancy ingredients. With lovely seasonal spiral vegetables, this dish is a treat for the tummy and visual eye candy. With simple ingredients and seasonal vegetable slow cooker ratatouille makes a perfect anti-inflammatory comfort food to enjoy on cold nights.

Prep time: 15 minutes, Cook time: 3 hours, Serves: 10

Ingredients:

- 2 large potatoes
- 1 medium sweet potatoes
- 1 red onion
- 2 red bell peppers
- 1 large yellow squash
- 1 green zucchini
- 3 cups marinara (homemade)
- 3 cloves garlic (minced)
- 1/2cup low-fat parmesan
- 1/2cup basil leaves
- Salt
- Pepper

Instructions:

1. Slice potatoes, sweet potatoes, and onions in 1/8inch thin rounds. Cut the zucchini and yellow squash in 1/2inch thin slices.
2. Pour one cup of homemade marinara sauce on the bottom of the slow cooker pot.
3. Place sliced veggies in a circular pattern, slightly overlapping each other. Follow this pattern: potato, sweet potato, zucchini, bell peppers, onion, and yellow squash. Repeat until you have used all the veggies.
4. After each row of veggies, sprinkle salt and pepper to taste. Also, add some minced garlic on over each row.
5. Pour the remaining sauce over the veggies and cook for 3 hours on high heat.
6. Garnish with basil and parmesan cheese before serving.

Notes: The recipe uses parmesan for garnish; you can use low-fat cottage, mozzarella, or parmesan for healthier options. Although mozzarella and cottage would taste fine with ratatouille parmesan, taste the best.

Nutritional Facts per Serving Size:

Calories: 329, Total Fat: 6.1g, Saturated Fats: 2.7g, Carbohydrates: 59.9g, Protein: 11.8g, Sugar: 18.4g, Fiber: 10.7g, Sodium: 447mg, Cholesterol: 10mg

Plant-Based Slow Cooker Chili

Tired of eating veggie-loaded salad but need your daily vegetable fix? Here is simple yet different vegan slow cooker chili recipe. The healthy nutrient-rich vegetables and beans in this dish are flavorful making a perfect zero-calorie anti-inflammatory meal for you.

Prep time: 20 minutes, Cook time: 9 hours, serves: 10

Ingredients:
- 2 medium yellow onion (chopped)
- 3 bell peppers 9red, yellow, green chopped)
- 3 cups pinto beans
- 6 large green jalapenos
- 2 can tomatoes (15 oz)
- 1 tbsp cumin powder
- 1 tbsp chili powder
- 2 tbsp oregano
- 1 tsp black pepper
- 3 bay leaves
- 1 tsp salt

Instructions:
1. Soak pinto beans overnight. Cover with water at least 3 inches deep.
2. Drain the beans and cook in the slow cooker with some salt. Add water and make sure it is 2 inches above the beans.
3. Cook on high heat for six hours.
4. After cooking, drain the beans and mix vegetables and other ingredients. Mix and cook for another 3 hours on high heat until beans have desired firmness.
5. Garnish with lime wedge and cilantro if you desire.

Nutritional Facts per Serving Size:
Calories: 326, Total Fat: 1g, Saturated Fats: 0g, Carbohydrates: 64g, Protein: 14g, Sugar: 6g, Fiber: 2g, Sodium: 508mg, Cholesterol: 0mg

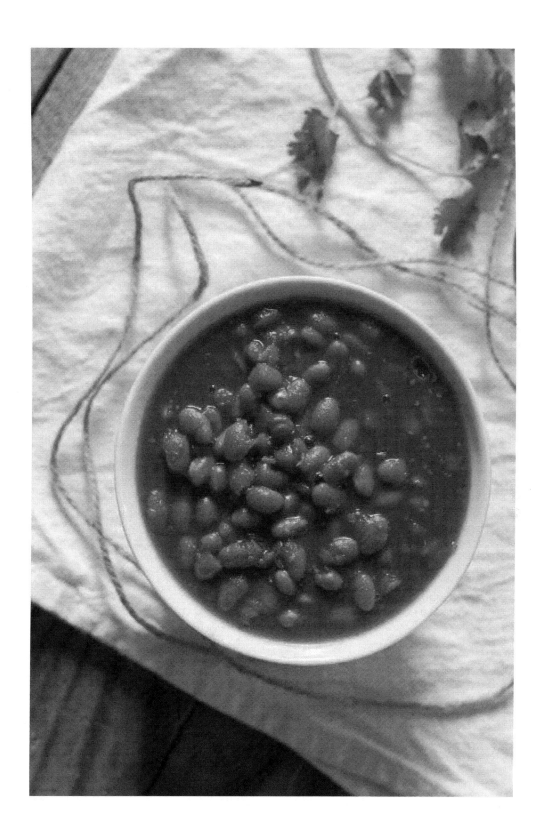

Beans and Legumes

Beans and legumes are the best foods to combat inflammation. Their anti-inflammatory qualities are unmatched. It is important to have most of your foods with salads, beans, grains, legumes, and fish when following an anti-inflammatory diet. Here are some yummy anti-inflammatory beans and legume recipes.

Slow Cooker Southern Style Green Beans

Southern-style green beans have never tasted so good. With this anti-inflammatory version of the recipe, you are going to fall in love with them. With eight hours of simmering in the slow cooker, green beans are nice and tender, just the way people love them in the South.

> Prep time: 15 minutes, Cook time: 8 hours, Serves: 16

Ingredients:

- 2 tbsp extra virgin olive oil
- 1 onion (diced)
- 2 cloves garlic (minced)
- 2lb green beans
- 1 tsp basil (chopped)
- 1 tsp black pepper
- 1 medium potato (chopped)
- 3 cups vegetable broth
- Salt to taste

Instructions:

1. Sauté onion and garlic in a medium skillet on low-medium heat for 4 minutes or until tender.
2. Add green beans, potatoes, vegetable broth, basil, pepper, salt, and sautéed onion and garlic in the slow cooker pot.
3. Cover and cook for 8 hours on low heat.
4. Serve with lemon wedges.

Slow Cooker Black Bean Soup for Two

Prep time: 5 minutes, Cook time: 6 hours, Serves: 2

Ingredients:

- 1 cup black beans (overnight soaked)
- 1 can diced tomatoes
- 1 cup vegetable broth (low sodium)
- ½ cup onion (diced)
- 1 clove garlic (minced)
- 1 carrot (diced)
- ½ cup sweet potatoes (diced)
- 1 cup baby spinach
- 1 mild green chili
- ½ tsp ground cumin
- 1/3 tsp ground coriander
- ¼ tsp red pepper flakes
- 3 tbsp chopped cilantro
- Greek yogurt for serving

Instructions:

1. Add all the ingredients in the slow cooker pot and stir.
2. Cover the slow cooker pot and set on low heat for 6-8 hours or until the carrots are tender.
3. Serve with a dollop of Greek yogurt.

Nutritional Facts per Serving Size (2 cups):

Calories: 299, Total Fat: 2g, Saturated Fats: 0g, Carbohydrates: 59g, Protein: 17g, Sugar: 12g, Fiber: 22g, Sodium: 607mg, Cholesterol: 0mg

Slow Cooker Red Lentil Curry

Lentils are the best anti-inflammatory foods to include in your daily diet. When it comes to cooking lentils, the possibilities are endless. Combined with spicy red curry, lentils would make a perfect meal. Red lentil curry is simply delicious and very easy to prepare in the slow cooker. Once all the ingredients are in the slow cooker, you will have your kitchen filled with the aromas of India. You can enjoy it with quinoa or brown rice. Your whole family will love this slow cooker recipe.

> Prep time: 15 minutes, Cook time: 6 hours, Serves: 8-10

Ingredients:

- 1 onion (chopped)
- 2 cups red lentils
- 1 clove garlic (minced)
- 1/2tsp cumin
- 1 tsp ground ginger
- 1/2tsp turmeric
- 3 tbsp red curry paste
- 2 tsp garam masala
- 4 tomatoes (chopped)
- 3 cups of water
- 1/4cup coconut milk
- Green onions (sliced)

For Garam Masala:

- 1/2tsp coriander
- 1/4tsp clove
- 1/2tsp black pepper
- 1/4tsp cardamom
- 1/4tsp cinnamon
- 1/4tsp nutmeg

Instructions:

1. Soak the red lentils at least fifteen minutes to half an hour before cooking.
2. Mix all the spices to make garam masala.
3. In the slow cooker pot, add onions, ginger, cumin, curry, paste, garam masala, turmeric, chopped tomatoes, and mix.
4. Drain the soaked lentils and add to the slow cooker pot.
5. Add 3 cups of water or more so that the lentils are covered with the liquid.
6. Cover the pot and cook for 6 hours on low heat until soft.
7. Add some salt and coconut milk before serving and mix.
8. Serve with quinoa or brown rice.
9. Garnish with fresh mint leaves.

Nutritional Facts per Serving Size:

Calories: 199, Total Fat: 2.9g, Saturated Fats: 1.3g, Carbohydrates: 31.4g, Protein: 12g, Sugar: 3.5g, Fiber: 14.4g, Sodium: 528mg, Cholesterol: 0mg

Slow Cooker Barbecue Beans

Slow cooker beans in barbecue flavor sound very tempting. But most barbeque beans are loaded with barbecue sauce in them, which has lots of sugar and preservatives making the beans anything but healthy. This recipe uses a healthier and cleaner version of barbecue sauce as it is homemade. Enjoy these slow cooker barbeque beans on their own or with brown bread

Prep time: 30 minutes, Cook time: 3 hours, Serves: 10

Ingredients:
- 2 cups Cannellini beans (soaked overnight or 4 hours)
- 1 onion (diced)
- 3/4 cup barbecue sauce
- 1/4 cup coconut sugar
- 2 tbsp yellow mustard
- 1/4 cup tomato sauce
- 1/2tsp black pepper
- 1/2tsp salt

For Barbecue Sauce:
- 1tbsp canola oil
- 1 onion (finely diced)
- 1 can tomato sauce (8oz)
- 1 clove garlic (minced)
- 1/4 cup organic vinegar
- 1/2cup mild sorghum or molasses
- 2 tsp Dijon mustard
- 2 tsp chili powder
- 1/2tsp cayenne pepper
- 1/4tsp black pepper
- 1/2tsp salt

For Garnish (optional):
- chopped parsley
- ground thyme

Instructions:

For Barbecue Beans:
1. In a medium saucepan, add canola oil and heat it on low, medium flame. Add onions and garlic, and sauté for 5 minutes.

2. Add the rest of the ingredients and stir.
3. Simmer for 30 minutes or until the sauce thickens.

For Beans:
4. Drain the water of soaked cannellini beans and add it to the slow cooker pot with the rest of the ingredients
5. Cover the pot and cook on low heat for 6-8 hours or high heat for 3-4 hours.
6. Garnish with thyme or freshly chopped parsley.
7. Serve with brown bread.

Note:
This recipe makes Barbecue sauce, which you can store in the refrigerator in a glass bottle or jar for up to a month. Use it in place of ketchup and other artificial sauces.
For beans, you can use pure molasses or raw honey if you do not have coconut sugar available. Honey is slightly sweeter than coconut sugar and molasses, so adjust accordingly.

Nutritional Facts per Serving Size:
Calories: 305, Total Fat: 3g, Saturated Fats: 0g, Carbohydrates: 57g, Protein: 17g, Sugar: 14g, Fiber: 12g, Sodium: 39mg, Cholesterol: 0mg

Sloppy Joes Made With Lentils

Here is another healthy Sloppy Joe recipe for you. This amazing Sloppy Joes recipe uses lentil and is so yummy you will not miss the beef. These sloppy joes with multi-grain buns are an ideal anti-inflammatory food fix; it is lip-smacking, nutritious, and vegan.

Prep time: 15 minutes, Cook time: 4 hours, Serves: 6

Ingredients:
- 2 cups brown/green lentils
- 4 cups of water
- 1 onion (chopped)
- 1 green bell pepper
- 2 cloves garlic (minced)
- 2 tsp mustard powder
- sucanat
- 1/2tsp chili powder
- 2tsp molasses
- 1 can (15oz) diced tomatoes
- 1 can (6oz) tomato paste
- 2 tbsp cider vinegar
- 1/4cup vegetable broth
- 1tsp salt

Instructions:
1. In a slow cooker pot place, garlic, bell pepper, lentils, and water. Cover the pot and cook for 3 hours on high heat or 6 hours on low heat.
2. Add mustard powder, molasses, sucanat, chili powder, vegetable broth, canned tomatoes, cider vinegar, tomato paste, and salt.
3. Cook on high heat for an hour.
4. Spoon the lentils on multi-grain buns or bread and enjoy.

Notes: For spicier lentil, Sloppy Joes substitute green bell pepper with two to three jalapenos.

Nutritional Facts per Serving Size:
Calories: 349, Total Fat: 2g, Saturated Fats: 0g, Carbohydrates: 67g, Protein: 20g, Sugar: 21g, Fiber: 24g, Sodium: 573mg, Cholesterol: 0mg

Slow Cooker Spanish Style Chickpeas

Chickpeas are loaded with fiber, proteins, and anti-oxidants. Any dish with chickpeas and the right blend of spices or dressing is fulfilling and delicious. This Spanish style slow cooker chickpea makes a yummy lunch or dinner in just a few calories.

Prep time: 12 minutes, Cook time: 4 hours, Serves: 6

Ingredients:
- 1 can chickpeas (15 oz)
- 3 tomatoes (diced)
- 1 onion (chopped)
- 2 potatoes (cubed)
- 2 cloves garlic (minced)
- 2 tsp smoked paprika
- 4 tbsp olive oil
- 4 cups of baby spinach
- salt to taste

Instructions:
1. Add chickpeas, tomatoes, onion, potatoes, garlic, paprika, and salt in a slow cooker pot. Stir well.
2. Cover the pot and set it to cook for 4-5 hours on low heat or until the potatoes are tender.
3. Add spinach and cook for 10 minutes until wilted. Stir halfway through.
4. Season with some olive oil, salt, and black pepper, and serve.

Notes: To make this meal more wholesome and fresh, use fresh and raw chickpeas instead of canned. All you need to do is soak the chickpeas the night before you cook them.

Nutritional Facts per Serving Size:
Calories: 330, Total Fat: 11g, Saturated Fats: 1g, Carbohydrates: 49g, Protein: 11g, Sugar: 18g, Fiber: 10g, Sodium: 758mg, Cholesterol: 0mg

The Ultimate 9-Bean Slow Cooker Soup

Save the best for the last! Here is the ultimate 9 beans slow cooker soup recipe. I know I have already given you enough soup recipes, but there is no such thing as too much soup, especially when you are on an anti-inflammatory diet and relying on your slow cooker.

With nine different types of fresh and dry beans, this healthy and hearty slow cooker, food is the ultimate comfort food. This recipe has black, kidney beans, split peas, pigeon peas, lentils, navy, lima, and navy. If you don't like certain beans, you can omit them and increase the quantity of the remaining ones. You can enjoy this 9-bean soup on its own or add a leafy green salad or hot crusty bread with it.

Prep time: 20 minutes, Cook time: 3 hours, Serves:8

Ingredients:
- ½ pound dried small kidney beans
- ½ pound dried lentils
- ½ pound dried navy beans
- ½ pound dried white lima beans
- ½ pound dried garbanzo beans
- ¼ pound dried green split peas
- ½ pound dried black beans
- ½ pound dried pinto beans
- ¼ pound dried pigeon peas
- ½ pound pearl barley
- 1 can (28oz) tomatoes (chopped)
- 1 turkey leg or mutton bone scrap
- 1 large onion (diced)
- ½ teaspoon rubbed sage
- 2 teaspoons lemon juice
- 1 teaspoon chili powder
- 1 teaspoon dried thyme
- 2 tsp salt
- ¼ cup small pasta (optional)
- ½ cup water

Instructions:
1. Soak white lima beans, navy, black, lentils, pinto, garbanzo, green split peas, pigeon pas, kidney beans and barley in water in a large pot. Cover the pot.
2. Before cooking, drain the beans and barley well.
3. Put beans, barley, water, turkey leg and scraps in the slow cooker, and bring it to the boil.
4. Cover the pot and simmer for 2 hours.
5. Add chili powder, thyme, sage, tomatoes, onion, and lemon juice to the slow cooker pot.
6. Add pasta and salt to the pot and cook for an hour on high heat.
7. Remove the turkey leg and de-bone the meat.
8. Chop the meat and add it back into the soup.
9. Serve hot and enjoy.

Nutritional Facts per Serving Size:
Calories: 299, Total Fat: 5g, Saturated Fats: 1g, Carbohydrates: 39g, Protein: 19g, Sugar: 5g, Fiber: 9g, Sodium: 450mg, Cholesterol: 17mg

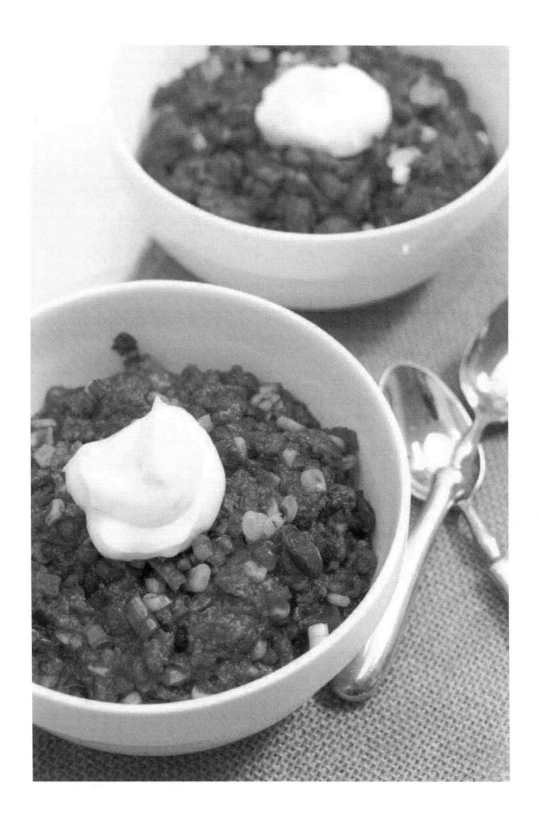

Poultry and Meat

While you are following a strict anti-inflammatory diet, I want to make sure you do not miss out on eating yummy dishes. That's why I gathered the best anti-inflammatory chicken and turkey recipes that you can easily prepare in a slow cooker for lunch or dinner. Some of these recipes are combined with fresh vegetables, whole grains, and low fat to make a lip-smacking meal for you.

Slow Cooker Turkey Chili

This easy slow cooker chili recipe has an amazing blend of turkey, beans, and chili, a perfect meal for all the spice lovers out there.

Prep time: 15 minutes, Cook time: 4 hours, Serves: 8

Ingredients:
- 1 tbsp vegetable oil
- 1lb ground turkey
- 2 cans Tomato soup (low sodium- 10.5oz)
- 2 cans black beans (15oz- drained)
- 2 cans kidney beans (15oz- drained)
- 1/2 medium-sized onion (chopped)
- 1 tsp red pepper flakes
- 2 tsp chili powder
- 1/2 tsp ground cumin
- 1/2 tsp garlic powder
- 1 pinch allspice
- 1 pinch black pepper
- Salt to taste

For garnish:
- Corn chips
- Sour cream

Instructions:
1. Heat oil in a skillet on medium heat. Cook turkey in the skillet until it is evenly brown.
2. Drain the turkey.
3. Coat the inside of the slow cooker or the liner with cooking spray.
4. Add in turkey, tomato soup, kidney beans, black beans, and onion.
5. Season with chili flakes, red chili powder, cumin, garlic powder, black pepper, allspice, and salt.
6. Cover the slow cooker and cook on high heat for 4 hours or low heat for 8 hours.
7. Serve with corn chips and a dollop of sour cream and enjoy.

Nutritional Facts per Serving Size:
Calories: 276 , Total Fat: 7.6g, Saturated Fat: 2.0g, Carbohydrates: 32.8g, Protein: 428g, Sugar:1g, Fiber: 11.3g, Sodium: 547mg, Cholesterol:420mg

Slow Cooker Black Bean and Chicken Chowder

Do not mistake chowder for soup. It is a thick chunky broth, which is either tomato or cream-based. This chowder is tomato-based and infused with Southwestern flavors.

Prep time: 5 minutes, Cook time: 4 hours and 30 minutes, Serves: 8

Ingredients:
- 3 chicken breasts (boneless and skinless)
- 1 cup frozen kernels
- 1 can black beans(low sodium, 15 oz, drained)
- 4 cups low sodium chicken broth
- 16 oz canned or homemade salsa
- 1/4 cup diced chilies

For garnish:
- 1/4 cup cilantro
- 1/2 cup avocado (sliced)
- 1 lime (cut into wedges)
- 1/4 cup yogurt

Instructions:
1. Add boneless chicken breasts, black beans, frozen kernels, salsa, and chilies in the slow cooker pot.
2. Pour the low sodium chicken broth in the broth and set the pot on low heat for 5-6 or high heat for 3-4 hours.
3. Remove the chicken when cooked and shred into pieces,
4. Put the chicken shreds back in the cooker and cook for 30 minutes on high heat.
5. Serve with yogurt, lemon wedge, and avocado slices.

Nutritional Facts per Serving Size:
Calories: 350 , Total Fat: 8g, Saturated Fat: 2.0g, Carbohydrates: 29g, Protein: 42g, Sugar:6g, Fiber: 9g, Sodium: 749mg, Cholesterol:100mg

Slow Cooker Spinach Artichoke Chicken

With creamy spinach and artichoke sauce, this chicken tastes like a gourmet dish. At the same time, it is very easy to make and is healthy too.

Prep time: 5 minutes, Cook time: 4 hours, Serves: 4

Ingredients:
- 8 cups spinach (chopped)
- 4 whole chicken breasts (bone-in with skin)
- 1 cup chicken broth
- 1 small onion (chopped)
- 3 cloves garlic (chopped)
- 4 tbsp cream cheese
- 4 tbsp parmesan cheese
- 6-8 artichokes heart
- 1 cup cherry tomatoes (chopped)
- Salt and pepper

Instructions:
1. Add chicken breasts, spinach and artichokes in the slow cooker
2. Pour the chicken broth into the pot. Add garlic, onion, salt, and pepper.
3. Cover the pot and set it to cook for 6-8 hours on low heat or 3-4 hours on high heat.
4. Stir in cream cheese and parmesan cheese into the pot before serving. The chicken will be covered in a creamy sauce.
5. Top with chopped cherry tomatoes to add nice visual and flavor before serving.

Notes: You can substitute 6-8 artichoke hearts with 14 oz preservative-free canned artichokes.

Nutritional Facts per Serving Size:

Calories: 246 , Total Fat: 6g, Saturated Fat: 2.0g, Carbohydrates:14g, Protein: 35g, Sugar:3g, Fiber: 4g, Sodium: 547mg, Cholesterol:82mg

Healthy Slow Cooker Chicken Dumplings

The way these light, pillowy dumplings float in a creamy chicken broth makes them the best comfort food for winter nights. With the goodness of whole wheat flour, these dumplings have no excess calories and a yummy chicken broth.

Prep time: 15 minutes, Cook time: 4 hours 30 minutes, Serves: 8

Ingredients:

- 2 chicken breasts (boneless and skinless)
- 6 cups chicken broth (low-sodium)
- ½ cup carrots (diced)
- ½ cup peas (frozen preferred)
- ½ cup celery (diced)
- 1 medium-sized onion (chopped)
- 3 cloves garlic (minced)
- 2 tsp dried thyme
- 2 tsp dried basil
- 1 tsp dried sage

For dumplings:

- 1/2 tsp garlic powder
- 1/2 tsp onion powder
- 3 tbsp. cold butter (cubed)
- 1 cup whole wheat flour
- 1 tsp baking powder
- 1/3 cup skim milk

Instructions:

1. Add chicken breasts, carrots, peas, onion, garlic, and celery in the slow cooker pot.
2. Add the seasonings, garlic, thyme, basil, sage and pour low sodium chicken broth in the cooker pot.
3. Set the pot to cook on low heat for 6 hours or high heat for 4 hours.
4. In a bowl, combine flour, butter, baking powder, onion powder, and garlic powder.
5. Mix the better in a way that the butter cuts into the dry ingredients. The mixture will turn into fine crumbs.
6. Add skimmed milk gradually until the mixture has a thick, batter-like consistency.
7. Remove the chicken from the cooker and shred into pieces. Add the shredded chicken back into the pot.
8. Drop the spoonful of batter into the pot. Make sure you don't make the dumplings too small, or else it will dissolve into the broth.
9. Cover and cook the pot for another 20 or 30 minutes on high heat.
10. Serve into the bowls and enjoy.

Note:

Prepare the dumpling batter before making this dish. This will allow the baking powder to produce gas bubbles that will give the dumplings a better texture.

You may not need to use the entire amount of milk or may need to use a little more.

Nutritional Facts per Serving Size:

Calories: 276 , Total Fat: 7.6g, Saturated Fat: 2.0g, Carbohydrates: 32.8g, Protein: 428g, Sugar:1g, Fiber: 11.3g, Sodium: 547mg, Cholesterol:420mg

Turkey Sloppy Joes

Sweet, messy, and lip-smacking sloppy joes are everyone's favorite. Unfortunately, they are a little unhealthy, and you can't enjoy them on the anti-inflammatory diet. But worry not, I have a healthier version of sloppy joes with whole-wheat, gluten-free buns to enjoy while sticking to your diet.

Prep time: 15 minutes, Cook time: 4 hours, Serves: 4-6

Ingredients:
- 1lb turkey breast
- ½ cup green pepper (diced)
- 1 medium-sized onion
- 3 cloves garlic (minced)
- ¼ cup homemade-sugar free or natural ketchup
- 1 tbsp yellow mustard
- 8 oz tomato sauce
- 1 tbsp BBQ sauce

Instructions:
1. Cook turkey breasts with onions and green pepper in a skillet over medium heat. You can skip this step and cook directly in the slow cooker, but it will give a better flavor.
2. Put the turkey meat, onions, and pepper in the slow cooker pot. Add minced garlic, ketchup, mustard sauce, BBQ sauce, and mix well.
3. Cover and cook on low heat for 3-4 hours or high heat for 2-3 hours. If you have not browned the meat in the skillet first, then cook on low heat for 5-6 or high for 3-4 hours.
4. Serve with whole wheat gluten-free buns.

Nutritional Facts per Serving Size (Bun not included):
Calories: 297 , Total Fat: 10g, Saturated Fat: 5g, Carbohydrates: 32g, Protein: 20g, Sugar:3g, Fiber: 4g, Sodium: 194mg, Cholesterol:32mg

Greek Lemon Chicken

This Greek Lemon Chicken slow cooker recipe is perfect for enjoying on weekends with your family.

Prep time: 5 minutes, Cook time: 4 hours, Serves: 4

Ingredients:
- 6-8 oz chicken breasts (boneless and skinless)
- 4 cloves garlic (minced)
- 3 tsp dried oregano
- 1/4 cup lemon juice
- 1 tbsp lemon juice
- 1 cup chicken broth
- 1 tsp salt

For garnish:
- 3 tbsp parsley (chopped)

Instructions:
1. Combine chicken breasts, garlic, onion, oregano, lemon juice and zest, chicken broth, and salt in the slow cooker pot.
2. Cover the pot and set the cooker on high heat for 4 hours or low heat for 6 hours.
3. Sprinkle with chopped parsley.

Nutritional Facts per Serving Size:

Calories: 253 , Total Fat: 2.0g, Saturated Fat: 2.0g, Carbohydrates: 15g, Protein: 24g, Sugar:8g, Fiber: 5g, Sodium: 1605mg, Cholesterol:97mg

Spinach-Chicken Meatball

If you think beef makes the best kind of meatballs, then you haven't tried spinach and chicken meatballs. Cooked with marinara sauce, spinach-chicken meatballs are perfect with zucchini noodles or squash spaghetti.

Prep time: 15 minutes, Cook time: 6 hours, Serves: 6 (makes around 12 meatballs)

Ingredients:
- 1 lb. chicken thigh or breasts (boneless)
- 1 large egg
- 1 tsp salt
- 2 tsp chili powder
- 2 tsp black pepper
- 3 cloves garlic (minced)
- 1 small onion (grated)
- 1/4lb baby spinach
- A handful of parsley (chopped)
- 2 tbsp olive oil
- 25 oz marinara sauce
- Spaghetti squash or zucchini noodle for serving

Instructions:
1. Combine ground chicken meat, egg, red chili powder, black pepper, and garlic in a mixing bowl.
2. Grate a small onion in the mixing bowl.
3. Finely chop parsley and spinach. Add spinach and parsley into the mixing bowl.
4. Mix well and roll into small 12 meatballs.
5. In a slow cooker, add olive oil and place the meatballs. Pour the marinara sauce over the meatballs and stir.
6. Set the cooker on low heat for 6 hours or high heat for 3 hours.

Nutritional Facts per Serving Size:
Calories: 167, Total Fat: 4g, Carbohydrates: 14g, Protein: 23g, Sugar: 8g, Fiber: 2g, Sodium: 387mg, Cholesterol: 420mg

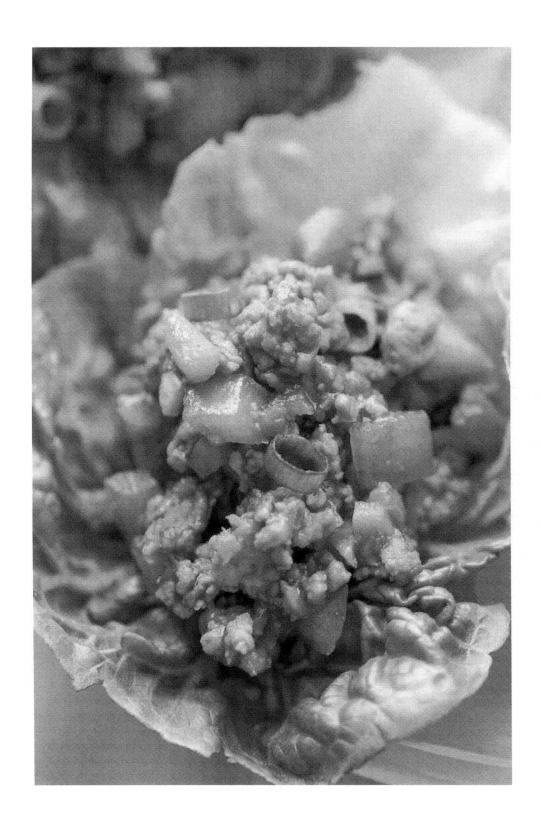

Beef Lamb and Pork

Most of the anti-inflammatory slow cooker recipes include soups, stews, and ones with vegetables and beans. But there is no rule saying that you cannot enjoy beef and other red meats when following an anti-inflammatory diet. You can enjoy beef once a week without disturbing your diet. Here are few anti-inflammatory recipes with beef, pork, and lamb; you can easily prepare in a slow cooker.

Korean Beef Lettuce Wraps

This delicious and fun way of eating wrap lets you enjoy beef with the goodness of lettuce.

Prep time: 10 minutes, Cook time: 8 hours, Serves: 8

Ingredients:
- 3 lb. beef (roasted)
- 6 cloves garlic (minced)
- 1 medium-sized onion (chopped)
- 1/3 cup Tamari sauce (gluten-free)
- 2 tbsp rice vinegar
- 2 tbsp sesame oil
- 1 tsp ginger (minced)
- 1/2 cup raw brown sugar
- 1/2 cup green onions
- 1/2 cup carrots (shredded)
- 8 lettuce leaves

For garnish:
- Slivered almonds
- Toasted Sesame seeds

Instructions:
1. Add tamari sauce, rice vinegar, brown sugar, oil, onions, and garlic in the slow cooker pot.
2. Add roasted beef in the pot and set it to cook on low heat for 8 hours.
3. When cooked, shred the beef with a fork. Drain the excess liquid and leave some to moisten the beef.
4. Take a lettuce wrap and add beef, diced carrots, and green onions. You can add silvered almond and toasted sesame seeds for flavor and crunch.
5. Serve and enjoy the lettuce wraps.

Nutritional Facts per Serving Size:
Calories:323, Total Fat: 10g, Saturated Fats: 3g, Carbohydrates: 16g, Protein: 23g, Sugar: 14g, Sodium: 64mg, Cholesterol: 105mg

Healthier Slow Cooker Texas Roadhouse Chili for Two

This healthy slow cooker chili is packed with tomatoes, beans, and meat, making it a perfect hearty dinner bowl for cold nights.

Prep time: 8 minutes, Cook time: 8 hours, Serves: 2

Ingredients:

- 1 ½ tbsp canola oil
- ¼ lb. ground turkey
- 1 cup fresh kidney beans (soaked overnight)
- 1 cup tomatoes (diced)
- 2 tsp chili powder
- ½ tsp garlic powder
- ¼ cup winter squash (diced)
- ¼ cup sweet potato (diced)
- ¼ cup carrot (diced)
- ½ cup water
- ¼ tomato juice
- pinch of red chili flakes (optional)

Instructions:

1. Heat oil in a skillet over medium heat. Cook ground turkey and onions in the skillet.
2. Cook till the meat is no longer pink.
3. Add meat, beans, tomatoes, diced vegetables, chili powder, garlic powder, water, and tomato juice in the slow cooker pot.
4. Set the pot to cook on 8 hours for low heat.
5. Add a pinch or two of red chili flakes if you want more spicy.
6. Pour into two serving bowls and enjoy.

Nutritional Facts per Serving Size (1/2 cup):

Calories: 324, Total Fat: 7g, Saturated Fat: 2g, Carbohydrates: 43g, Protein: 25g, Sugar: 9g, Fiber: 2g, Sodium: 200mg, Cholesterol: 39mg

Slow Cooker Pork Tenderloin

This lean and juicy slow-cooked pork tenderloin is very easy to make. All you need to do is marinate the pork tenderloin overnight in the fridge and let the slow cooker do its work the next day.

Prep time: 10 minutes, Cook time: 8 hours, Serves: 8

Ingredients:
- 3-4lb pork tenderloin

For Marinating:
- 1 cup chicken broth (low-sodium)
- 1 tbsp rice vinegar
- 1 tbsp Dijon Mustard
- 1 tbsp soya sauce
- 2 cloves garlic (minced)
- 1 tbsp fresh ginger (grated)
- 1/2 tsp black pepper
- 1 tsp curry powder
- Salt to taste

For Glaze: (optional)
- 2 tsp soya sauce
- 2 tsp raw honey
- 2 tbsp rice vinegar
- 2 tbsp ketchup
- 1 tablespoon Dijon Mustard
- 1 tbsp sesame oil

Instructions:
1. In a large mixing bowl, combine all the ingredients for marinating the pork.
2. Trim the fat off of the pork tenderloin and cut into 2-inch pieces. Coat the pork tenderloin pieces with the marinade evenly and refrigerate overnight.
3. Add the marinated pork tenderloin in the slow cooker and cook on low heat for 4-6 hours until the pork can be easily shredded.
4. To prepare the glaze, add all the ingredients in a small saucepan and mix. Bring it to boil and reduce the heat to simmer for five minutes or until the glaze has the desired thickness.
5. Put the pork tenderloin on the serving plate and pour the glaze over it.

Nutritional Facts per Serving Size:
Calories: 252, Total Fat: 2g, Saturated Fat: 0g, Carbohydrates: 15g, Protein: 32g, Sugar: 18g, Fiber: 0g, Sodium: 387mg, Cholesterol:74mg

Slow Cooker Moroccan Beef Stew

Traditional Moroccan flavors and anti-inflammatory spices make this dish ideal for all the beef lovers out there. The beefy stew is warm, fragrant, and has the goodness of fresh vegetables.

Prep time: 15 minutes, Cook time: 6 hours, Serves: 6

Ingredients:

- 1 1/2 lb. beef stew cubes or chuck roast cubes
- 1 ½ tbsp extra virgin olive oil
- 3 tbsp whole-wheat flour
- 3 garlic cloves (minced)
- 1 tsp black pepper
- 1/4tsp ground cumin
- 1/4tsp turmeric
- 1/4tsp red chili flakes
- 1 tsp paprika
- 1 tsp cumin
- Salt to taste
- 1 yellow onion (coarsely chopped)
- 2 celery stalks (diced)
- 2 carrots (diced)
- 2 tomatoes (diced)
- 1/2cup beef broth

For garnish:

- ¼ cup silver almonds
- ¼ cup raisins

Instructions:

1. Cut beef into cubes and cover in whole-wheat flour. Heat oil in a skillet and cook beef cubes for 5 minutes or until brown.
2. Transfer beef into the slow cooker. Add all the remaining ingredients and stir. Cover the pot and cook for 6-8 hours on low heat.
3. After the cooking time, add raisins and almonds. Cook for another 10 minutes on high heat.
4. Serve the stew on its own or add couscous or brown rice.

Notes: You can freeze the beef stew for up to 2 months.

Nutritional Facts per Serving Size:

Calories:339, Total Fat: 12g, Saturated Fat:3g,Carbohydrates: 32g, Protein: 29g, Sugar: 19g, Fiber: 5g, Sodium: 558mg, Cholesterol: 73mg

5–Ingredient BBQ Pulled Pork for Two

If you love southwestern food, but you are avoiding fatty foods, then you can enjoy this BBQ slow cooker pulled pork guilt-free. This recipe swaps out fatty pork shoulder for lean pork chops, and sugary BBQ sauce with a homemade healthier BBQ sauce. This recipe only uses 5 ingredients, so there is no reason you shouldn't try this one.

Prep time: 15 minutes, Cook time: 6 hours, Serves: 6

Ingredients:
- 12lb lean boneless pork loin chops

For BBQ Sauce:
- 1/2 tsp apple cider vinegar
- 4 oz no-salt tomato sauce
- 1 tbsp raw honey
- 1/2 tsp adobo sauce (plus 1 chipotle pepper for spicier flavor)
- Kosher salt and pepper to taste

Instructions:
1. To make the BBQ sauce, mix all the ingredients except the pork loin in a slow cooker pot. If you want a spicier BBQ sauce, add in a chipotle pepper with the adobo sauce. For a milder BBQ sauce, just the adobo sauce will work fine.
2. Put pork loin chops into the sauce and set the cooker on low heat for 4-6 hours or high heat for 2-3 hours, until the internal temperature of the meat reaches 165 degrees.
3. Serve and enjoy.

Nutritional Facts per 1/2cup Serving Size
Calories:383, Total Fat: 16g, Saturated Fat:5g,Carbohydrates: 24g, Protein: 37g, Sugar: 21g, Fiber: 2g, Sodium: 5716mg, Cholesterol: 117mg

Low Carb Beef Stroganoff

When you walk in the door after a long day, the smell of beef stroganoff welcomes you, and you are all set to enjoy this delicious, low-carb, anti-inflammatory meal. Instead of pasta, this beef stroganoff combined with cauliflower, green beans, and broccoli makes a good wholesome meal.

Prep time: 15 minutes, Cook time: 6 hours, Serves: 4

Ingredients:
- 1 onion (chopped)
- 2 garlic cloves (minced)
- 2 slices bacon (chopped)
- 1lb beef stewing steak (cubed)
- 8 oz mushrooms
- 1 cup broccoli heads (florets)
- 1 cup cauliflower heads (florets)
- 1/2cup green beans
- 3 tbsp tomato paste
- 1 tsp smoked paprika
- Salt to taste
- 1 cup beef stock
- Sour cream for serving (optional)

Instructions:
1. Place onion, garlic, chopped bacon, beef cubes, mushroom, vegetables, spices, and salt in the slow cooker pot.
2. Pour beef broth into the pot — cover and cook for 6 hours on low heat.
3. Serve with sour cream if desired.

Nutritional Facts per Serving Size:

Calories:317, Total Fat: 19g, Carbohydrates: 8g, Protein: 29g, Sugar: 4g, Fiber: 1g, Sodium: 558mg

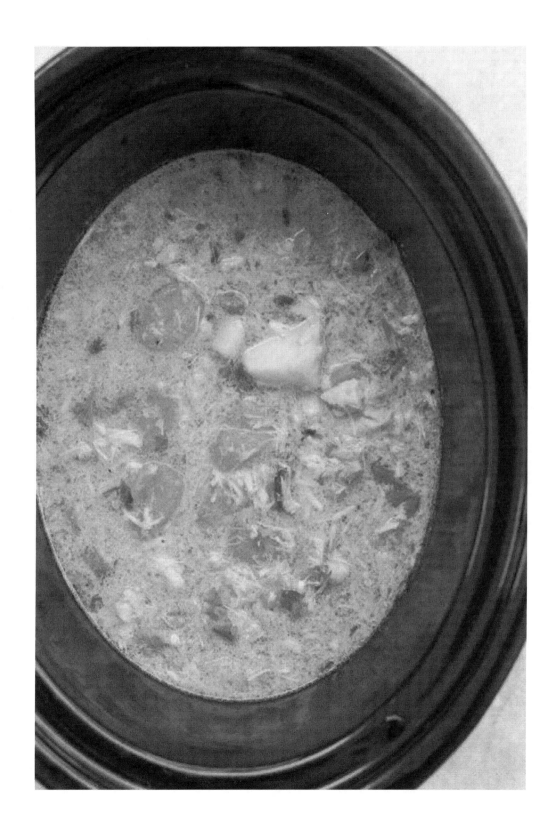

Fish and Seafood

By now, you must know how good fatty fishes are for an anti-inflammatory diet. Fishes are the best source of protein if you're following an anti-inflammatory diet. Fishes like sardines, mackerel, salmon, and tuna are packed with Omega-3 fats and anti-oxidants. These fishes lower inflammation, protects the heart and helps reduce bulging waistline when taken at least twice a week. Here are anti-inflammatory fish meals to keep you fit.

Slow Cooker Salmon with Creamy Lemon Sauce

This salmon recipe is easy to make and is big on flavor, tenderness, and juiciness.

Prep time: 10 minutes, Cook time: 2 hours 20 minutes, Serves: 6

Ingredients:
For Salmon:
- 3 lemons
- 1 1/2 lb. skin-on salmon
- 1/2 tsp paprika
- 1/2 chili powder
- 1 tsp Italian seasoning
- 1 tsp garlic powder
- 1 tbsp lemon juice
- 1 cup low sodium vegetable broth
- Salt and pepper to taste

For Creamy sauce:
- 3 tbsp lemon juice
- 1/4 cup chicken broth
- 2/3 cup low fat cream
- 1/8 tsp lemon zest
- parsley (for garnish)

Instructions:
For Salmon:
1. Place a large piece of parchment paper in the slow cooker pot.
2. Cut lemons into slices and arrange the layer of sliced lemons in the middle of the slow cooker pot.
3. Place salmon on top of the lemon slices. Spray some cooking spray on the salmon.

4. Season the salmon with paprika, chili powder, garlic powder, Italian seasoning, salt, and pepper. Rub all the seasonings all over the salmon with your fingers.
5. Pour lemon juice and vegetable broth in the slow cooker pot around the fish, DO NOT pour over the fish.
6. Set the cooker on low heat for 2 hours.
7. Preheat the oven to 400 degrees.
8. If your slow cooker can handle heat up to 400 degrees, then pop it in the oven to get the browning top of the salmon for 5 -8 minutes. Or else transfer the salmon onto your oven tray or baking tray.
9. Take out the fish from the oven and transfer it to the cutting board. Set the fish aside.

For Creamy Sauce:
1. In a small saucepan, add lemon juice, broth, and low-fat cream on medium heat.
2. Reduce the heat to low and cook for 8 minutes with the lid closed.
3. Add in lemon zest and cook on high heat for 2 minutes or till the sauce thickens and reduces.

Serve:
4. Cut the salmon into individual fillets.
5. Plate up the fillet with creamy lemon sauce and chopped parsley.

Notes: For the sauce, instead of fresh lemon juice, you can use the lemony broth from the cooked salmon as well.

Nutritional Facts per Serving Size:
Calories:304, Total Fat: 19g, Saturated Fats: 7g, Carbohydrates: 7g, Protein: 31g, Sugar: 1g, Fiber: 1g, Sodium: 240mg, Cholesterol: 119mg

Orange-Chipotle Shrimp in Butter Lettuce Cups

Now here is a very fun anti-inflammatory shrimp recipe for you. You will not only enjoy eating it but making it too. This recipe has an awesome blend of shrimp, chipotle chilies, and tangy orange. It is light, refreshing, and makes a perfect meal to fill your tummy with.

Prep time: 10 minutes, Cook time: 1 1/2 hours, Serves: 6

Ingredients:
- 4 oranges
- 2 lb. peeled shrimp
- 1 bunch asparagus
- 3 tomatoes (diced)
- 2 tsp chopped chipotle chilies in adobo sauce
- 2 tbsp olive oil
- 2 tbsp tomato paste
- 1 tsp red pepper flakes
- 16 butter lettuce leaves
- 1/4cup chopped cilantro or parsley (fresh)
- 2 avocados (diced)
- Orange zest

Instructions:
1. Zest the oranges first.
2. Remove the white fiber of the orange and cut the slices in half. Set aside.
3. In a slow cooker pot, add shrimps, orange zest, asparagus, diced tomatoes, tomato paste, red chili flakes, olive, and chipotles. Toss well.
4. Set the cooker to cook on high heat for 1 ½ hour or until the shrimps are cooked well.
5. Put the lettuce leaves on the serving platter. Add shrimps, orange segments, avocado, and parsley.

Nutritional Facts per Serving Size:
Calories:310, Total Fat: 12g, Saturated Fats: 4g, Carbohydrates:12g, Protein: 27g, Sugar: 8g, Fiber:8g, Sodium: 244mg, Cholesterol: 172mg

Crockpot Halibut Stew

Other than Omega-3 fats, Halibut is rich in essential proteins, Potassium, Selenium, and Vitamin B12. Stew is not the first thing that comes to mind when you are thinking of cooking Halibut. But there are plenty of great seafood stews to make for an anti-inflammatory diet.

Prep time: 5 minutes, Cook time: 8 hours, Serves: 6

Ingredients:
- 1 small yellow onion (coarsely chopped)
- 1 red bell pepper (diced)
- 1 large potato (cubed)
- 2 carrots (thinly sliced)
- Juice of 1 lime
- 1 ½ cup Chicken broth or Vegetable broth
- 2 cloves garlic
- 1 tsp chili powder
- ½ tsp black pepper
- ½ tsp red pepper flakes
- 1 tsp cumin
- 1/4 cup cilantro (finely chopped)
- Salt to taste
- 1lb halibut filet (bite-size pieces)

Instructions:
1. In a slow cooker pot, add onion, potatoes, carrots, bell peppers, lime juice, broth, garlic, cilantro, and all the seasonings. Set the pot on low heat to cook for 8 hours.
2. Add halibut fillet and set the pot to cook for 30 minutes on high heat.
3. Garnish with more cilantro if desired and serve.

Notes: You can substitute halibut with other fish.

Nutritional Facts per Serving Size:
Calories:148, Total Fat: 2g, Saturated Fats: 1g, Carbohydrates: 12g, Protein: 18g, Sugar: 4g, Fiber: 2g, Sodium: 296mg, Cholesterol: 26mg

Slow Cooker Fish and Tomatoes

Prep time: 10 minutes, Cook time: 2 ½ hours, Serves: 4

Ingredients:
- 1 lb. fish
- 15 oz diced tomatoes
- 1/3 cup vegetable broth (low sodium)
- 1 bell pepper (diced)
- 1 small onion (diced)
- 1 garlic clove (minced)
- 1 tsp dried parsley
- 1/4 pepper
- 1/2 tsp salt

Instructions:
1. In a slow cooker pot, add onions, bell peppers, garlic, and diced tomatoes. Add fish of your choice and stir.
2. Sprinkle salt, pepper, and parsley on the top of fish.
3. Pour the broth on the top.
4. Cover and set the pot to cook for 1-2 hours on high heat or 2-4 on low heat.
5. Serve.

Nutritional Facts per Serving Size:

Calories:152, Total Fat: 19g, Saturated Fats: 0.8g, Carbohydrates: 8g, Protein: 25.2g, Sugar: 4.5g, Fiber: 1.3g, Cholesterol: 56.3mg

Slow Cooker Italian Herb Salmon

Prep time: 5 minutes, Cook time: 2 hours, Serves: 6

Ingredients:
- 1 lb. salmon
- 1 bell pepper (diced)
- 1 small onion (diced)
- 15 oz diced tomatoes
- 1 garlic clove (minced)
- ½ tsp fresh herbs (thyme or sage)
- 1 tsp Italian seasoning
- ½ tsp salt

Instructions:
1. Add onion, peppers, tomato broth, Italian seasoning, garlic, and salt in the slow cooker pot. Mix well and set the pot to cook for 1-2 hours on high or 2-4 hours on low.
2. Add salmon and fresh herb. Cook for another 30 minutes on high heat.
3. Serve hot and enjoy. You can also serve with cauliflower rice or brown rice.

Nutritional Facts per Serving Size:
Calories:196, Total Fat: 5.5g, Saturated Fats: 1g, Carbohydrates: 9g, Protein: 26, Sugar: 2.8g, Fiber: 1.6g, Cholesterol: 57.9mg

Healthy Slow Cooker Tuna Casserole

This slow cooker casserole cannot be any easier. This healthy casserole has whole-grain noodles and homemade cream of mushroom soup, making an amazing tuna casserole you will never forget after you have it once.

Prep time: 20 minutes, Cook time: 1 1/2 hours, Serves: 8

Ingredients:

For Cream of Mushroom:
- 1 cup white mushroom (sliced)
- 2 tsp olive oil
- 3 cup chicken broth (low sodium)
- 2 cup almond milk
- 1 tbsp vinegar
- 1/4 cup whole wheat flour

For Casserole:
- 4 cups whole-grain noodles
- 2 cups mixed vegetables (mushrooms, carrots, zucchini or anything you like)
- 2 cans of tuna (28 oz)
- 1 garlic clove (minced)
- 1 tsp pepper
- salt to taste

Instructions:

1. To make the cream of mushroom soup sauté mushrooms in oil until they turn a little brown.
2. Add vinegar and whole wheat flour to the mushrooms and stir.
3. In a large pot, add mushroom mix, chicken broth, and almond milk. Bring it to boil and simmer on low heat for 8-10 minutes.
4. Let the soup cool down a bit,
5. In a slow cooker pot, add cream of mushroom soup, vegetables, whole-grain noodles, tuna, salt, pepper, and garlic.
6. Stir and cover the pot. Set the put to cook on high heat for 1 ½ hour or low for 3 hours.
7. Let the casserole cool down for a bit as it will be too hot to eat.
8. Serve and enjoy.

Nutritional Facts per Serving Size:

Calories:171, Total Fat: 1g, Saturated Fats: 0g, Carbohydrates: 27g, Protein: 11g, Sugar: 1g, Fiber: 2g, Sodium: 269mg, Cholesterol: 17mg

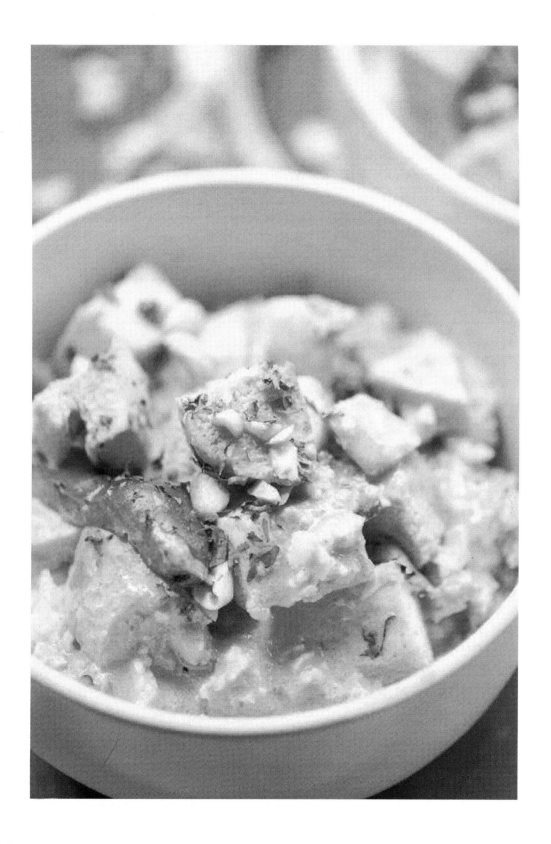

Desserts

If you think you cannot enjoy deserts when on anti-inflammatory diet, you are so wrong. Here, I have amazing slow cooker desert recipes that are not only low-carb and low-fat but taste as good as the regular deserts. Make sure to include the desserts in your meal plan while taking care of your calorie count.

Slow Cooker Fudge

This recipe is to fulfill your insatiable chocolate cravings. While you are avoiding your favorite bar of chocolate, enjoy this decadent and guilt-free chocolate fudge which you can easily make in your slow cooker.

Prep time: 15 minutes, Cook time: 3 hours, Serves: 20 chocolate fudge pieces

Ingredients:
- 2 ½ cup dark chocolate chips
- ¼ cup coconut sugar
- ½ cup coconut milk
- 2 tbsp coconut oil
- 1 tbsp vanilla extract
- Dash of salt

Instructions:
1. In a slow cooker pot, add chocolate chips, coconut milk, coconut sugar, coconut oil, and salt and stir.
2. Cover the pot and cook for 2 hours on low heat.
3. After cooking, remove the lid and add vanilla. Do not stir the fudge at this point. Allow cooling at room temperature. Take help of a candy thermometer and see when it reaches 110 degrees.
4. When cooled, use large spoon and stir vigorously for 5-10 minutes until the mixture loses its glossiness.
5. Oil a glass tray or pan with a little bit of coconut of olive or coconut oil. Pour the fudge in the tray and refrigerate for 4 hours or until the fudge hardens.

Nutritional Facts per Serving Size:

Calories: 114, Total Fat: 8g, Saturated Fats: 4g, Carbohydrates: 17g, Protein: 1g, Sugar: 10g, Fiber: 1g, Sodium: 21mg, Cholesterol: 0mg

Pumpkin Pecan Cobbler Recipe

This dish combines the two classic fall flavors to give you a warm and delicious dessert. Enjoy the gooey pumpkin peach cobbler made in slow cooker.

Prep time: 15 minutes, Cook time: 3 hours, Serves: 8

Ingredients:

For Filling:

- 1 cup whole wheat flour
- 2 tsp baking powder
- ½ tsp salt
- ¾ cup coconut sugar
- 2/3 cup pumpkin puree
- 1 ½ tsp pumpkin spice
- ¼ cup coconut milk
- ¼ cup butter
- 2 tsp vanilla

For topping

- ½ cup coconut sugar
- ½ tsp vanilla
- ¼ tsp cinnamon
- 1/3 cup diced pecans
- 1 ¾ cup boiling water

Instructions:

1. Spray the inside of the slow cooker pot with non-sticking oil spray.
2. Whisk all the dry ingredients in a mixing bowl.
3. In a separate bowl, mix together the remaining wet ingredients of the filling.
4. Combine the dry and wet ingredients and whisk until the filling is slightly thickened.
5. Pour the batter evenly in the slow cooker pot.
6. Whisk the topping ingredients in a mixing bowl and pour over the filling. Set the pot to cook on high heat for 2-3 hours or until the top layer browns.
7. Serve and enjoy.

Nutritional Facts per Serving Size (1/2 cup):

Calories: 318, Total Fat: 10g, Saturated Fats: 0g, Carbohydrates: 56g, Protein: 2g, Sugar: 46g, Fiber: 2g, Sodium: 236mg, Cholesterol: 15mg

Slow Cooker Lemon Bars

Want a light lemony fulfilling desert? These slow cooker lemon bars are a must to try.

Prep time: 15 minutes, Cook time: 3 hours, Serves: 12 lemon bars

Ingredients:

For Crust
- 1 ½ cup whole wheat flour
- ½ cup oat flour
- 1 tbsp lemon zest
- 1 tbsp coconut sugar
- 2/3 cup coconut oil
- ½ tsp salt
- Ice cold water

For Filling
- 2 large eggs
- 8 oz low-fat cream cheese
- ½ tsp vanilla
- ½ tsp coconut sugar
- 1 tbsp lemon zest
- 2 tbsp lemon juice
- ½ cup flour
- ¼ tsp salt
- 2 ½ cup blueberries

Instructions:

For crust
1. Combine all the ingredients of crust except ice cold water and work it with your hands until crumbly.
2. Slowly add ice water, two tablespoons at a time until a dough consistency is achieved.
3. Form dough ball and store inside an airtight container in the fridge for half an hour.

Filling
4. Beat cream cheese on high setting and gradually add in eggs and beat.
5. Add the rest of the ingredients and beat. Do not over-beat.
6. Fold in blueberries with a rubber or silicone spatula.
7. Spray slow cooker and line the bottom with the dough and then add filling on top.
8. Cook for 2-3 hours on low heat until the edges brown.
9. Wait to cool and cut into square bars.

Nutritional Facts per Serving Size (1 bar):

Calories: 319, Total Fat: 19g, Saturated Fats: 11g, Carbohydrates: 81g, Protein: 7g, Sugar: 14g, Fiber: 3g, Sodium: 240mg, Cholesterol: 81mg

Slow Cooker Chocolate Peanut Butter Cake

Enjoy the rich combination of chocolate and peanut butter in this healthy and decadent recipe of chocolate cake.

Prep time: 15 minutes, Cook time: 4 hours, Serves: 16

Ingredients:
- 1 cup whole wheat pastry flour
- 1 tbsp baking powder
- 2 egg whites
- ½ cup coconut sugar
- 2 tsp pure vanilla
- 1/3 cup peanut butter
- ½ cup cocoa powder
- ¾ cup apple sauce

Instructions:
1. Line the bottom of the crockpot with a parchment paper and spray the inside.
2. Combine the dry ingredients in a mixing bowl. Combine wet ingredients in a separate bowl and beat until thick. Pour wet into the dry ones.
3. Stir until all ingredients are combined.
4. Pour in the slow cooker and set to cook for 4 hours on low heat or until a knife comes clean.
5. Cut into pie-like pieces and serve.

Nutritional Facts per Serving Size:
Calories:141, Total Fat: 3g, Saturated Fats: 2g, Carbohydrates: 19g, Protein: 3g, Sugar: 10g, Fiber: 3g, Sodium: 440mg, Cholesterol: 0mg

Slow Cooker Hot Fudge Cake

Prep time: 15 minutes, Cook time: 3 hours, Serves: 8

Ingredients:

Cake:
- ¾ cup coconut sugar
- 1 cup whole wheat flour
- 2 tsp baking powder
- ¼ tsp salt
- ¼ cup melted butter
- ½ cup dark chocolate chips

Hot Fudge Sauce:
- ¼ cup of cocoa powder
- ¾ cup coconut sugar
- 1 tsp pure vanilla
- 1 ¾ cup boiling water

Instructions:
1. Spray the cooker with non-stick oil.
2. Whisk dry ingredients except for chocolate chips and wet ingredients into separate bowls. Combine the ingredients and beat until the batter thickens.
3. Combine hot fudge ingredients and mix.
4. Sprinkle chocolate chips on top and pour the hot fudge sauce.
5. Cook for 3 hours on high heat.

Nutritional Facts per Serving Size:

Calories: 60, Total Fat: 3g, Saturated Fats: 0g, Carbohydrates: 7g, Protein: 18g, Sugar: 4g, Fiber: 2g, Sodium: 440mg, Cholesterol: 0mg

Almond Rice Chia Pudding

This almond rice and chia pudding is a pure treat to anyone who loves dessert but wants to maintain a healthy diet.

Prep time: 15 minutes, Cook time: 3 hours, Serves: 6

Ingredients:
- 2 cups brown rice
- ½ cup raisins
- 5 cups almond milk
- 3 tbsp chia seeds
- 1 cinnamon
- ½ cup honey

Instructions:
1. Add all the ingredients in a slow cooker and stir.
2. Cover and cook for 2-3 hours on high heat.
3. Sprinkle some chia seeds when serving.

Nutritional Facts per Serving Size (3/4cup):

Calories: 366, Total Fat: 4g, Saturated Fats: 2g, Carbohydrates: 69g, Protein: 12g, Sugar: 4g, Fiber: 1g, Sodium: 451mg, Cholesterol: 15mg

Made in the USA
San Bernardino, CA
15 February 2020

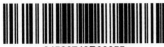